Peaceful Dying

Peaceful Dying

The Step-by-Step Guide to Preserving Your Dignity, Your Choice, and Your Inner Peace at the End of Life

DANIEL R. TOBIN, M.D.

with

KAREN LINDSEY

PERSEUS BOOKS
Reading, Massachusetts

Many of the designations used by manufacturers and sellers to dis-
tinguish their products are claimed as trademarks. Where those designations appear in this book and Perseus Books was aware of a
trademark claim, those designations have been printed with initial
capital letters.

FairCare is a trademark of the FairCare Health System.

Library of Congress Catalog Card Number: 98-88126

ISBN 0-7382-0034-4

Copyright © 1999 by Daniel R. Tobin, M.D.

Perseus Books is a member of Perseus Books Group

Cover design by Suzanne Heiser
Text design by Joyce C. Weston
Set in 12-point Minion by Pagesetters Inc.

123456789-DOH-0302010099
First printing, November 1998

Perseus Books are available at special discounts for bulk purchases in
the U.S. by corporations, institutions, and other organizations. For
more information, please contact the Special Markets Department at
HarperCollins Publishers, 10 East 53rd Street, New York, NY 10022,
or call 1-212-207-7528.

Visit us on the World Wide Web at
http://www.aw.com/gb/

*To everyone who supported the creative processes
that made this work possible.*

*To all the living teachers who, in their time and
beyond, have passed on wisdom and inspired
goodness through their actions.*

*To the realization of the potential master
in each and every one of us.*

Contents

Contents

Introduction

O UR SOCIETY is currently awakening to the special needs of the dying. We are finally developing the will to confront dying and to help those who have entered this very important part of life. Too often people do not have the support they need in facing the personal issues that surround death. *Peaceful Dying* has been written for people who want the practical tools to make that happen. Throughout, this book highlights the relation between understanding the nature of peaceful dying and searching for meaning in life: peaceful dying is as much about living well as it is about dying well.

Although everyone would agree that peaceful dying is a human right, it can be very hard to arrange. Many studies have borne out what people experience over and over again: the current medical system too often lacks the training and perspective to offer patients a peaceful, comfortable end of life. The Institute of Medicine's comprehensive publication *Approaching Death: Improving Care at the End of Life* demonstrates the need to change a health care system that allows "too many people to suffer from pain and other distress that clinicians could prevent or relieve." A study published in the *Journal of the American Medical Association* has found that many patients die in moderate to severe pain and that living wills are often ignored.*

---

* Institute of Medicine, Committee on Care at the End of Life, *Approaching Death: Improving Care at the End of Life*, ed. Marilyn J. Field and Christine K. Kassel (Washington, D.C.: National Academy Press, June 1997); The Support Principal Investigators, "A Controlled Trial to Improve Care for Seriously Ill Hospital Patients," *Journal of the American Medical Association* 277, no. 20 (November 22, 1995).

The problem goes far beyond simply a medical one. Indeed, modern medicine has the tools to make dying at least physically comfortable; there are many medications that can alleviate the pain people might experience. The fact that so often these tools aren't used speaks to a far deeper problem—the denial of death itself, by the public at large and by the medical profession. When you avoid facing death, you can't do the work necessary to reach peaceful dying.

And it *is* work. It's a bit like climbing a steep mountain. To make the final ascent, you need a lot of preparation and effort. Just because dying is natural doesn't mean it's easy. Having some level of guidance and counseling as you proceed through this work can help a lot.

I became aware of the importance of peaceful dying early in my medical career. From the beginning of medical school, I was disturbed by the training I *wasn't* getting; there was no formal instruction in caring for the dying, in my medical school or in any others I knew of. In addition, we were being taught to see dying as a disease and death as the doctor's failure to cure that disease. But I could accept that only in a very limited way. Certainly it was important to stop people from bleeding to death and to give the right treatment or medication when a life could be saved. It made sense to forestall death when a patient could be given comfortable years or months of life. But I knew that death was inevitable for all of us and that the time of dying needed to be recognized and honored. Why was the simple fact that we all die being ignored? I felt the failure in medical philosophy deeply, and I knew very early on that I wanted to develop a new system for caring for the dying and an educational program to teach this system once I had developed it. As a senior medical student in 1982, I began working with one of the first U.S. hospices. I have remained active in end-of-life education and health care delivery ever since.

Introduction

Although I entered a surgical specialty, in 1995 I began concentrating most of my energies on end-of-life educational training, working with the dying at the VA Medical Center in Albany, New York. Since that time I've worked with hundreds of dying patients. I immersed myself in this work in part because I wanted to help people who were dying and in part because, through working with them, I could gain the knowledge and experience that would help me create the system I knew was needed. This was to be a comprehensive, reproducible, and flexible model that would empower people in their own end-of-life situations.

I researched all the programs I could find. The hospice movement has created a system for helping people at the end of their lives. The British Macmillan cancer nurses, a palliative-care team trained to care for cancer patients and their families, was the closest to the system I envisioned, but I learned from all the models I studied.

Through my work at the VA center, where I was a palliative-care physician and hospice consultant, I created the FairCare Health System, a physician-based consultant unit that provides education, counseling, advocacy, and coordination of services for people facing end-of-life situations. And I began to create and refine the twenty-six steps that constitute the system for peaceful dying that I call FairCare. This book takes the reader through the program's steps. It is directed primarily to those who are currently facing end-of-life situations and secondarily to their loved ones. The text of each step includes practical suggestions and illustrations from the experiences of dying patients I have worked with. Some steps will not be meaningful to some readers: that's fine. If there's a step that doesn't interest you, feel free to skip it and move on.

Dying isn't a disease, but a natural part of life. It shouldn't be "treated" with endless procedures that serve only to create terrible discomfort and perpetuate an illusion that with enough machines we can defeat mortality. Once you know the specifics involved in end-of-life situations and acquire the knowledge and communication skills to discuss them, it becomes possible to shift from a predominantly cure-based medical treatment to a care-based system, if that is what you want.

Sadly, much of the public has come to see "a good death" as synonymous with "assisted suicide." *Peaceful Dying* focuses instead on accepting the naturalness of dying while taking advantage of the medications that can make the pain most people dread obsolete.

Our culture's emerging recognition of the importance of peaceful dying will create a demand for and openness to programs that help people die with dignity and comfort. A culture that routinely uses methods of peaceful dying will in time see that such programs have a strong effect on the entire community. Nowhere is the opportunity for teaching and incorporating wisdom and compassion into our communities greater than in our treatment of the dying.

Whenever I work with people in end-of-life situations, I am struck by the extremes of the human experience. The emotions of dying are intense, difficult, and varied. But they are not necessarily terrible; indeed, sometimes they are incredibly beautiful, and even at times extremely happy. I always consider how our culture's overwhelming fear of death blots out that reality: we rarely achieve a whole view of dying, which encompasses every emotion and which, as I'll demonstrate throughout this book, can be profoundly positive.

I have great respect for traditional medicine and its practitioners, the doctors and nurses whose lives are spent trying to heal people. But the limitations of their training often keep fine health care workers from being helpful to their dying patients. At the same time, the public's fear of dying and the tendency of many patients to request drastic treatments in a vain effort to defeat death have created an unhealthy situation. It is time for mainstream medicine to take on the work of meeting the physical, emotional, and spiritual needs of dying patients as part of routine health care. It is my hope that the FairCare concepts will help bridge the gap that so often exists between doctors and patients in end-of-life situations. If this can be achieved, the living that you do throughout your dying can be, if you let it, some of the most meaningful and joyful living you've ever experienced. I hope this book helps you to live that kind of dying.

PART ONE

A Look at the Dying Process

CHAPTER 1

Dying as a Natural Part of Living

My Journey to This Work

*A*s a third-year medical student in 1982, I was assigned to a medical team caring for a tall, frail, eighty-eight-year-old man who was dying of multiple diseases, all very advanced. When I walked into his room, Mr. Arnold* was curled on his bed in the fetal position, staring blankly toward the ceiling. It was clear that he did not have much longer to live.

"Mr. Arnold," I said gently, "I'm Doctor Dan Tobin. I have to ask you a few things."

Politely but apathetically, he struggled to answer my questions. "I'm going to draw some blood now," I told him after I'd finished with my forms. "We have to do a few tests on you." His chart indicated that several specialists, including those for heart, kidneys, and gastrointestinal tract, were scheduled to perform tests on him. At first he seemed confused; then he looked at me and said, very clearly, "Please, no more tests on me. Please, I beg of you, everything has been tested. All I want to do is go home. Please send me home."

Trying to sound confident, but in fact unsure of what was right, I replied, "But we have to take these tests in order to help you."

"Please," he repeated. "Please, no more tests." His eyes were sunken, red rimmed, sad, and full of fear. His fear was not of

---

* I have changed the names of all my patients to protect their families' privacy.

death, but of me and what I was about to do him. He wanted to go back to Parry Rest Nursing Home, where he lived, to die in peace. It was a simple request made by one human being to another. But he knew that I would refuse this request and that I would participate, along with all the other doctors, in making his final days a nightmare wracked with pain.

For six days, doctors performed various tests. The gastroenterologist passed tubes up and down both ends to search for tumors. The respiratory specialists were taking blood gases—an extremely painful blood test in which the blood is taken from the arteries in the wrist. The primary care doctors ordered daily blood tests to determine medication changes. Finally, Mr. Arnold's heart gave out. A full-scale code blue, the all-out effort to resuscitate a patient, was initiated. I stood in the corner of his hospital room and watched the senior staff pump stimulants into his veins, then place a large intravenous catheter into his neck. An eager and strong young doctor ripped open Mr. Arnold's hospital gown, placed his hands on the old man's chest, and began vigorously pumping his entire upper body. I listened as his ribs cracked under the hands of the muscular young resident. Then came the machines. First a breathing mask with a hand pump forced air into Mr. Arnold's lungs. Then a clunky breathing machine called a ventilator was rushed into the room, and someone threaded a breathing tube into his mouth and down his windpipe. His chest heaved as the machine pumped oxygen into his lifeless lungs. Electrical paddles were placed on his chest. I watched his body jump off the bed with each application of the electrical paddles.

I stood in that corner trying to contain an explosion of conflicting emotions—sadness, anger, and confusion. I could not reconcile the remarkable contradiction between what the doctors, nurses, and technicians were doing and what this man wanted. Were these people doing all this because they thought it was right? *Was* it right? I wanted to know. I worried about what we would do next if the old man survived this episode. What condition would he be in? Would we do yet more painful, useless tests on him? None of us could possibly have any illusions that we could make him well again. Whatever we did, he would soon die. All our machines and all our tests could do nothing but make him suffer in the little time he had remaining.

The team tried to revive Mr. Arnold for ten minutes, but his body did not respond. Reams of electrocardiograph paper splattered with the old man's blood covered the floor, every inch of it testimony to the obvious: he was dead. Finally, the senior physician called off the code blue. Respiratory therapists, five doctors, three nurses, and three medical students all looked down at the floor, dejected. They had failed in the one thing their training had told them mattered—they had not prevented death. I too felt that we had failed Mr. Arnold, but in a very different way. As the doctors and therapists filed out of the room and the nurses started to clean up the body and disconnect the machines and fluid lines, I found a note on the floor, written by this old man.

> Everything has been Tested
> I was told I was going to being tested
> I hope to go to Parry Rest
> to day.
>
> Please let me go
> to day
>
> no more Tests on me
> for any thing

I knew that dying didn't have to be that way. It did not have to be an impersonal event mediated by cold technology. I had seen the importance of peaceful dying at a very early age. When I was eight, I'd spent a lot of time in my uncle's home, where my ailing great-grandfather lived. I knew he was dying, but it didn't scare me. Everyone treated it as natural. I was deeply impressed by the local family doctor, who routinely made house calls and who tended to my great-grandfather's dying. He was a tall, slender man, elegant and very distinguished. An Italian immigrant, Dr. Minetta brought the old country ways with him, making house calls regularly.

The doctor's visits were a major event in the family. Everything quieted down; a sense of awe permeated the house as he examined my great-grandfather. There was a feeling of tranquillity on these occasions. We'd look at each other and think, "It's all right, Dr. Minetta is here." It wasn't false hope that he gave us. He never suggested that Great-Grandpa was not going to die; he simply made death seem less terrible. He was gentle with the dying man; he listened to him; he gave him medications to dull the pain. He never asked that the other children and I be sent away. We were part of the family, part of Great-Grandpa, and it was right that we should be part of his dying. I felt a kind of hero worship for Dr. Minetta and decided that I too would one day be a doctor. Partly it was because of all the attention he got. Someday, I thought, everyone would become quiet when I walked into a room. They would all stare at me with awe and wring my hand with gratitude. It was a grand fantasy for an eight-year-old. But equally, and ultimately more importantly, I wanted to help people the way he did. His compassion struck me deeply—so deeply that it remains etched in my mind to this day.

Yet when I went to medical school, I discovered that we weren't trained to face dying as calmly as Dr. Minetta did. People with advanced illness were dying without guidance. There was no organized system of caring for them. Nowhere in all my training was there formal instruction in caring for the dying, in the nature of dying, or in how a patient's dying affected the health care practitioner. I was shocked by how many people were left to die alone, suffering physical and emotional pain. Large teams of academic physicians and physicians in training, along with nurses and other health care practitioners, concentrated on curing disease, rarely making sure the patient understood all the available treatment options.

I saw the fears patients had about their illness and the discomfort of the practitioners in the face of those fears. The doctors seemed to be fighting the dying process to the bitter end. Patients would request that everything be done to keep them alive, without being told that nothing could be done to keep them alive for more than a few days or weeks and that many of the life-prolonging techniques would be hideously uncomfortable. Families too would beg the doctors to do anything possible to keep their loved ones from dying. I found it hard to watch people request all the advanced technological medicine. I recall vividly the fear and pain in the eyes of many patients who were holding onto every moment and not receiving assistance with the emotional aspects of their dying. Many of the people I began my clinical and medical experience with were dying in pain and terror.

Most of the doctors I worked with appeared unable to accept dying as a natural progression of living. To the physicians and the staff, death was seen as a defeat, and a patient's dying was often referred to as a personal failure. The doctors seemed overburdened, worried about their patient load and the possibility of malpractice suits. Most of them appeared uncomfortable talking with patients—or even with medical colleagues—about dying. Further, they usually hadn't developed the interpersonal skills required to fully relate to dying people. Only a few of the physicians were able to talk comfortably about their dying patients and indeed about themselves—the emotional difficulties involved in becoming and being a physician. None of their training had addressed how those feelings would affect their approach to dying patients.

There were exceptions. I recall several great doctors who were comfortable in caring for the dying and who took the time to explain the importance of learning these skills to their students. These few men and women were humble, worldly, and quite skilled as clinicians. They taught me that the medical system greatly affects people's lives, and especially their dying. These doctors knew how to listen to their patients: they routinely sat at patients' bedsides, expressing concern for their needs. They went out of their way to be available to the families and loved ones of their patients. They were acutely aware of the suffering, both emotional and spiritual, that their dying patients went through, and they were always attentive to such suffering. They never forgot a dying patient's humanity.

In the early years of my medical practice, I strove for a way to reconcile the contradiction I kept seeing between the physicians' passion to relieve pain and the pain we routinely inflicted on our dying patients. As I searched for my own place within medicine, I was lucky enough to have a broad medical experience. I worked for a while in a remote, rural part of the country, then at large and prestigious university teaching hospitals. I spent two and a half years providing medical services in the predominantly poor, African American neighborhood of Harlem in New York City. Very early on I was struck by one common theme among the patients I worked with: however different they were in other ways, all had similar experiences and needs at the time of death. The wealthiest and the poorest, the Ph.D.'s and the barely educated all experienced death in very similar ways. As I progressed in my career, I worked in a number of different disciplines, not all of them medical. At different times I worked as a waiter, career counselor, creative manager in the music business, developer of children's cartoon characters, director of a foundation addressing childhood hunger in the United States, general physician, eye surgeon, and hospice palliative-care physician. I worked with and got to know many different types of people with many different cultural backgrounds and beliefs. As I worked in these various professions, I was always pulled by the experiences I had had with dying people, and the sense of how each individual's struggle formed the essence of the human condition. Eventually the power of these experiences and my desire to help people in the last stage of life led me into hospice palliative-care medicine, where I began working in 1995. As a medical student and an intern, I had been powerless to prevent the suffering inflicted on the dying. I knew, finally, that my focus in medicine must be to help reverse the attitudes that had created so much needless suffering and deprived so many people of good and peaceful deaths.

I have been working with the dying ever since. Initially, I simply wanted to offer physical and emotional comfort, to provide pain relief, and to answer medical questions that might come up. But gradually I found my role expanding as I learned more and more about what people needed at this stage of life and what they were capable of experiencing. Eventually I realized that, like all other stages of life—infancy, puberty, adolescence, adulthood, and old age—dying offered unique opportunities for growth, understanding, and spiritual awakening. I began to integrate this realization into my work.

The History of Medicine in Relation to the Dying Process

To understand our current medical system and its potential for helping people, as well as the current practice toward the dying person, we need to look briefly at some basic history of medicine. Throughout documented history there has always been some form of medical practice, which, until the last fifty years, involved a healing art with limited technical resources. All Eastern and Western practices of medicine were originally based on a concept of preventing illness, helping the person's body heal by responding to disease, and administering to the suffering of people with a great sense of care. Prompting the body to heal itself when possible, as well as creating a quiet mental state, were valued ideals.

A spiritual component to understanding the relationship between illness and healing has existed throughout the history of medicine. Spirituality, for our purposes, is defined as a person's individual understanding of, and relationship to, a higher power, a vital source of energy, and eternity. Spirituality often leads to an appreciation of some form of celebration as a regular part of living. Integration of what is now called mind-body medicine, the understanding that emotions can affect disease as well as healing and wellness, is seen throughout the evolution of medical philosophy. Historically, great emphasis was placed on caring for the emotional needs of the dying person and understanding that dying well meant dying in good spirits whenever possible.

During the mid-1600s, in the age of enlightenment, science began to distance itself from a holistic approach to disease. In the mid-1800s, the germ theory, the theory that microbes caused disease, was developed. The opposing view at that time was that the body's system weakened, allowing microbes to grow in what would be called an opportunistic state. With the advancement of antibiotics in the 1930s, medicine could prevent the spread of infectious diseases. It also began to make great strides in curing diseases. Soon thereafter came the development of vaccines. Families began bringing their dying to hospitals. Dying became institutional, changing our relationship to it dramatically.

As technology advanced, medical instrumentation, X rays, and an abundance of diagnostic and therapeutic treatments allowed for rapid advances in medicine and surgery. Many life-saving instruments and techniques were routinely employed in medical practice, and the acute medical model for treating and curing disease became a part of mainstream health care. Modern medicine quickly achieved excellence in managing medical emergencies, including trauma, heart attacks, infections, and many other conditions. However, the marriage of technology and medicine has resulted in significant problems in the areas of caring for the dying person.

Perhaps the greatest limitation of Western medicine has been its refusal to acknowledge the inevitability and naturalness of death, and how important a part of life it is. The passion to pro-long life and to enhance it is wonderful, to a point. It is probably responsible for most of the great advances of modern medicine. But when it doesn't take into account the simple fact that at some point life can't, and shouldn't, be prolonged, it creates, rather than alleviates, suffering. If we in medicine cannot accept dying as a natural part of living and embrace the dying process, we neglect people when they are most vulnerable, most alone, and most desperately in need of love, comfort, and a very specific kind of care. With the best of intentions, we sometimes inflict on our patients treatments that are extremely painful, and we neglect their real needs.

Over the last fifty years, U.S. medicine has blossomed into a giant business, currently surpassing a trillion-dollar-per-year cost. Many significant trends, including the creation of fee-for-service delivery of health care, have caused the system to change dramatically. As this system becomes transformed into a new managed-care model (expanded from employers providing health care for their employees), people find themselves at the bottom of an inverted pyramid trying to figure out how to secure good-quality health care. As a result of many different pressures within the health care delivery system, the doctor-patient relationship is becoming seriously challenged, exacerbating the difficulties in end-of-life care. The doctor-patient relationship is historically based on intimacy, trust, and the belief that the best medical decisions regarding treatment will be made. To rebuild the relationship, the public must be able to see a change in the way in which doctors manage end-of-life situations on an individual basis.

Fortunately, our society is beginning to realize that there is a natural time to die, that at some point the body and mind are ready to stop fighting. Yet although there has been an increased awareness of the dying process and of the need for peaceful dying, studies show that few hospitals create conditions for peaceful dying and that living wills are too often ignored. Too many people have died isolated, fearful, and in physical and emotional pain. Too many families have endured lonely, frightening days and nights watching their loved ones dying. With some guidance, much of this suffering can be alleviated. As a result, today there is a great public outcry for a system of medical care that can help people make choices in dying and have those choices honored.

We need a formula that can help people know what to talk about throughout the process of dying and how to get the right professional help with these issues. We need a comprehensive system to help dying people, their families, friends, and medical providers communicate about the dying process. Most of all, we need to recognize that peaceful dying can be defined by specific criteria and that it is something most of us would want for ourselves and for those we love if given the chance. To achieve peaceful dying, it's important to learn how to talk about dying and how to empower oneself to fight for it.

It's useful here to look at how the women's health movement has fought for, and sometimes won, changes in Western culture's approach to birthing. For many decades, doctors dictated the specifics of obstetrical care and women were instructed to give birth in a specific manner. Women were ordered to stay in bed, usually anesthetized, and kept from participating in the birth of their children. Although that is still sometimes the case, it's no longer the norm. Today women often deliver children in positions they request, in handsomely decorated delivery suites, surrounded by loving family and friends. Fathers who used to wait outside the room during the birth of a child are now welcome participants in the process. Sometimes close friends or relatives also assist in the birthing process. The number of women who give birth at home has increased, and many are turning to the original health professional for childbirth, the midwife. Once the initial shift in consciousness developed, economic forces pushed great changes in the business of obstetrical care as women began demanding these new (or, rather, old) approaches.

We can learn a lot from this. Just as the women's health movement has succeeded, to a degree, in changing the way we treat childbirth, restoring it to a more natural approach, so we can all participate in shifting the way the current medical system treats dying. The demand for compassionate, natural caring needs to be implemented as the standard of care in medicine when people decide they are ready to die.

Dying: The Benevolent Teacher

As I began working with different people in their end-of-life situations, I found that the process of dying was a powerful instructor. I saw that dying was an intense and unique period of life, a transition of unparalleled magnitude. A great deal of growth and understanding developed for people as they approached their dying. I discovered that, in most cases, the search for meaning in life was intensified by the dying process. Everyone who faced dying at some point began asking such questions as,

"What is really the meaning of my life?" "What have I done with my life?" and "What does our life mean anyway?" It was at this time that I made an amazing discovery—the wealth of personal introspection and healing that could be learned from examining the dying process.

The reality of death is a living truth that takes root within us early on. As soon as we become aware of change, we become aware of death. Children learn about dying when their pets die. As we age, we see the deaths of grandparents, then of parents. As our own bodies pass from young adulthood into middle age, and further into old age, we see the signs of our own mortality. Though each of us deals with the reality of death differently, the fact that we will die serves as a living teacher, shaping our lives and the way we treat ourselves and others, for good or ill. When people are dying they reflect on their lives, and in their private moments they think about their lot in life. Dying invariably creates a wider awareness of life. This doesn't mean that everyone becomes kinder or more sensitive: much depends on the type of person involved. In some cases, fearing death itself, people become more selfish, lashing out at the world that seems to be abandoning them.

In my experience, though, this situation is rare. Lying in bed, with time to think, most people do soften, and spend time reviewing their lives. For those who are able to contemplate and accept death, there often comes an increased recognition of how essential love, honesty, and forgiveness are for being at peace with oneself. In some cases, the awareness of death makes people more focused and determined; in others, it mellows them and makes them more tolerant.

One of my patients was a middle-aged woman who had led a busy life, raising five children and living the life of a socialite. She had never been particularly introspective. Now she had metastatic ovarian cancer and had to lie, inactive, in a hospital bed.

We spent many hours talking about her life. She felt that she had lost a lot by not being more reflective. Over time, she began to realize that much of her bustling activity had served as a means of avoiding personal reflection. Always in motion, she had rarely caught a glimpse of her deepest feelings. Now, forced to stay in bed, she was also forced to reflect. She realized that she had failed to listen when her children had tried to communicate that they needed more emotional attention than she offered. She spoke of this regretfully, but felt she had reached in her dying a depth and reality in herself that her busy life had never afforded her. She began the process of making peace with her children. I did very little active counseling with this woman; all I provided was the space in which she could do the reflecting she so desperately needed to bring her life to a peaceful close.

Another patient of mine had been abusive to his wife and children. He was a tough, elderly man, tattooed from head to toe. Now he was dying of prostate cancer. Our hospice's social worker contacted his children, telling them their father was dying and this was their chance to say good-bye. They refused to come. At first he was angry, but as we talked he began to evaluate his life. He realized that he had been wrong, and spoke often to me of his longing to be forgiven. He began to read poetry, something he would previously not have allowed himself to do: he found in the words of the poets an expression of his own longing to be understood.

Searching for Meaning

All the people I have worked with through their dying have reflected on the meaning of their lives in their own individual manners. I usually encourage people to ask questions about their lives. Most are able to ask and answer questions about life's meaning when they've done this. Asking yourself questions allows you to confront your fear of dying and of what does or doesn't come after it: the fear of nonexistence lies at the core of the denial of death. Simply thinking about your dying for a few moments and reflecting on your impermanence, which is one of life's certainties, can help lessen the fear. Often people come to believe that there is life beyond this life or that there is a kind of immortality in the work and love they have left behind. Looking at your dying can be one of the greatest catalysts for growth. Dying can be welcomed and viewed as a great friend. Throughout life, contemplating death can nurture the values that support life.

During the dying process, the spiritual truths that underlie life can emerge with irrefutable clarity. It's as if the lessons we were learning the slow way throughout life suddenly become distilled and intensified when we start to die. Once people enter the dying process, they often see the necessity of love, forgiveness, letting go of resentments, and making peace with those who accompanied them through life. Dying people who embrace these values achieve a kind of serenity that has often eluded them during their lives. Unfortunately not everyone does embrace these values. Some hold onto bitterness, as power driven in dying as they were in living. Though they see the chance for change, they reject it, often showing extreme spite toward the people around them. In so doing, they also lose the serenity that they might have discovered in their last days.

What I have found with many of my patients is that from the dying process can emerge a kind of generic spirituality, consisting of universal truths that are common in all religions. This doesn't occur only with those who have been involved in specific religions; sometimes the least religious people are the most spiritual.

Death isn't just a benevolent teacher to the dying. The living too, if they allow themselves to be part of a loved one's dying, learn valuable lessons—lessons that can enrich their lives and in turn offer strength to their own dying when it comes. It's not always easy to see this at the time, when grief and loss are all-consuming. It usually takes time and the diminishing of the pain to see what growth has occurred as a result of the participation in a loved one's dying.

It can be especially difficult when the dying person is a child, yet I've seen even that tragedy teach valuable lessons to the survivors. A dying child can give incredible gifts to a family and loved ones. I learned this early in my medical training, with a nine-year-old girl named Jamie. She was on a hospital ward, dying of leukemia. When I first introduced myself to her, Jamie sensed how uncomfortable I was. She immediately tried to reassure me. "Doctor Dan," she said, "I'm okay with all that's going on. I've been in and out of the hospital for the past three years, and I know I'm going to die and go to heaven." Amazed by her calmness and her maturity, I spent as much time as I could with her and her family. I began to see that Jamie's role in the family was that of caretaker: she was teaching them, with her own ease, that dying wasn't so terrible. "I'm okay," she'd constantly reassure them. "It's all really okay."

Jamie's mother had great difficulty accepting the final days of the girl's dying. "Remember me," Jamie would ask her, and all the rest of us who clustered around her. "Remember the good times we had; remember me with love." Her mother tried as well as she could, but it was her father who really took in the lesson. At first tight-lipped, he said to me, "If she accepts her dying, I guess I have to." But he soon grew beyond that, coming not only to acceptance but to genuine peace. During her last few weeks, Jamie gave away all her favorite objects—to her parents, her sisters, the staff members she had grown close to. She taught everyone that her dying could not be negotiated away and that she was at peace. "Just remember me," she asked us. It's been many years, but certainly I still remember Jamie, and I am certain everyone else involved in her dying does too.

Treating the Living and Caring for the Dying

Many people argue that we should fight death completely, even at the very end of life, because only by making such a determined struggle can we ever hope to keep the living alive. From this perspective, refusing any possible life-prolonging treatment is a form of suicide; for a doctor to stop treating a person's disease, no matter how advanced it may be, is a form of murder.

But this is a sad distortion of what medicine is about. Certainly, prolonging life is important—when there really is life to prolong. Unless you are killed by an accident, a sudden heart attack, or a stroke, chances are very good that you will develop some life-threatening illness—cancer or a disorder of the lungs, heart, kidneys, or liver. Such diseases are very often treatable and sometimes even curable, particularly if they are detected in their early stages. At this point, it makes sense for you to do everything you can to stay alive and for your doctors to do all they can to save you.

But sometimes these diseases do not get cured, no matter when they are detected. The illness progresses until all treatment options have been exhausted, and you've reached the turning point when the disease process has become the dying process. Your eventual death will not be your doctor's failure or your own, but a natural end to physical existence.

One of the things I've seen over and over as I've worked with dying patients is that there almost always comes a point, well before a person dies, when the doctor or the patient—or both—realizes that the illness has progressed beyond any medical hope of recovery. Most people who have been stricken with a life-threatening illness know they are going to die, even when their doctors have kept such information from them.

One of my patients, a fifty-three-year-old man who contracted liver cancer and went through several rounds of chemotherapy, told me how he had come to understand that he would die soon. "I looked up toward the heavens and simply asked, 'Why?' " he said. "The next thing I heard were the words, 'Because it's your time.' I knew from that moment on that I was going to die. I had never spoken to God before, and he had never spoken to me, but I knew that was him talking to me then. After that, I stopped the treatment. It was just a matter of getting ready."

This man had realized in his own way what his oncologist could have told him: that further treatment would have been pointless because liver cancer, especially in its advanced stages, is usually incurable. He died twenty-two days later.

Another of my patients, a fifty-nine-year-old laborer, had cancer of the mouth and throat. His tumor grew into a mass the size of a softball on the right side of his jaw. Eventually, we knew, it would block blood flow to his brain and bring on a fatal stroke. Surgery was impossible, and after several rounds of chemotherapy and radiation, none of which slowed the tumor's growth, the man decided to stop all treatment. His medical team had told him that he had between four and six months to live, and he decided he didn't want to make that period any more painful than it already was. All he wished to do at that point was to be with his family and prepare for his death.

A self-educated man, he had read a great deal about various religions. One day while the two of us were sitting together, he started to talk about what he was facing. "I'm going to go on living," he said to me. "But I will live on as energy in heaven. Right now, I'm paying for some of my mistakes."

"What do you mean?" I asked.

"Some people believe there's a purgatory in the afterlife. I don't believe that," he said. "But I do believe that dying is a kind of purgatory. It's a way of letting go of stuff you don't need, and getting ready for the next stage of life."

For both these men, further treatment would have been not only futile, but inhumane. It would not have changed the outcome of the disease but certainly would have altered the quality of what remained of their lives.

Such is the case with the vast majority of people whose physical lives are ended by disease. Once the turning point has been reached, further treatment of the disease not only contributes to physical and emotional suffering, but often prevents people from making peace with their lives and preparing for what lies ahead.

Mainstream medicine can learn much from the early work in the field of thanatology and the groundbreaking efforts of the worldwide hospice movement—Cecily Saunders in the United Kingdom, Elisabeth Kubler-Ross in the United States, and all the people who have paved the way for hospice care to be integrated into our health system. The hospice philosophy embraces meticulous attention to pain control, as well as the importance of addressing the patient's psychological and spiritual needs in dying. Hospices developed the understanding that it may be desirable to stop attempts to cure disease when death is approaching and inevitable. It thus pioneered the concept of death with dignity and humane pain management. It is time to move to a next stage, in which palliative care is incorporated throughout the fabric of mainstream medicine.

When I was a senior medical student, I met Dr. N. Michael Murphy, a general physician and psychiatrist who had recently begun a hospice in Albany, New York, where I was training. This was pioneering work, as there were few hospices in the United States at that time. Dr. Murphy brought the tradition and art of caring for the dying into medical practice while facing a significant amount of resistance from the medical establishment. Few doctors would refer their patients to his hospice, which they saw as unnecessary and interfering with the hospitals' work. Dr. Murphy's hospice team began practicing and teaching a type of medicine based on a person's right to die in peace. Fortunately, the increasing public demand for processes that allowed death with dignity forced the medical establishment to become less resistant to hospices, and the hospice movement has seen a significant growth over the past several years.

In his work Dr. Ira Byock, a hospice pioneer, has emphasized the importance of improving and measuring the quality of life in dying.

What we need now is to take what the hospice movement has done and expand it, so that people can die in hospitals, homes, and hospices with the same level of comfort and care. We also need to do more to help people with advanced disease, and their health care workers, understand the psychological issues of facing dying at a much earlier stage, and in greater depth, than the traditional hospice program has achieved. When we provide this level of quality standardized care, we will have paved the way for peaceful dying to be within everyone's reach.

CHAPTER 2

The Human Response to Dying

*I*N COUNSELING many people with terminal illnesses and participating in their peaceful deaths, I have observed distinct stages through which they pass on their way to death. From the moment a person hears the diagnosis of an end-of-life disease to the moment of death, there is a real and natural timeline. Its length varies from person to person, since the length of time between diagnosis and death varies greatly with different diseases and different people. Nevertheless, in my experience, the stages usually follow the timeline.

If you have been diagnosed with an end-of-life disease, you may find it helpful to see yourself as being at the very beginning of a new phase of life. You'll progress through physical, psychological, and spiritual stages of great struggle and growth. The growth can be difficult, but if you work with it, it can bring you understanding and peace.

You can help make this happen by trying to distance yourself for a time, watching your own life as if you were an outside observer. Look at everything. Rather than focusing on just one issue in a given situation, consider how the events of your life lead to one another and affect one another. Look at living and dying from a perspective of wellness and disease if you can. Until now, your body was able to fight off illnesses because of its natural defenses—what I call the natural balance of wellness, when the body can return to wellness and balance out disease.

Now this has changed. Understand that there is a healthy way to face reality and a natural balance of wellness that may integrate into fighting your disease. Most people go through shock, and they grasp at life, trying to cure the illness. That makes sense. But it helps to realize that your natural balance of wellness has been severely altered by your disease and that you're embarking on an effort to restore that balance. This will take time and effort. Though there may be remissions, or even a cure, there's no magic bullet.

Drawing on my own experience with patients as well as on the work of Dr. Elisabeth Kubler-Ross and others, I have articulated six common reactions that a person facing an end-of-life diagnosis experiences after hearing the prognosis: shock, grasping, grief, letting go, healing, and serenity. Each of these is a distinct emotional and psychological condition. Several can exist simultaneously, but one or another will dominate the person's consciousness at various points of the dying process. These reactions are a natural human response to facing the harsh reality of an end-of-life disease. They are best understood as emotional and spiritual states of being, rather than as completely distinct stages. Often they overlap. Shock is usually followed by grasping and grief, but most people will move back to these first three reactions even when experiencing aspects of healing and letting go. Often people spend a lot of time in the stages of grasping and grief, without realizing they are in shock over their diagnosis. You don't need to label each emotional reaction you are having, but the awareness that these six reactions exist can help you understand your response to what's happening with you.

Shock

Your first reaction will probably be shock. Despite the endless litany of metaphors for the impact that a prognosis of dying has on a patient, no description can adequately communicate the trauma. You are desperate to look away from this truth. Shock, a protective mechanism, is a natural response; it allows you to deal with the meaning of your doctor's words in digestible portions.

One of the patients I counseled was Sandra, a fifty-year-old woman with advanced cervical cancer. A socially active and free-spirited woman, Sandra had avoided doctors: her cancer was detected only when she had been admitted to a local hospital with severe stomach pain. In all our initial conversations, Sandra insisted that the diagnosis must be wrong—despite the biopsies that proved otherwise. It took several weeks for her to admit what was happening to her, to move on to discuss her grief and sadness, and to begin exploring decisions about her treatment and about the remainder of her life.

Along with shock, you'll experience fear. Both are coping mechanisms, but fear is a sign that you're facing the truth and dealing with it as best you can. What most people fail to realize is that, in time, fear can be controlled and even diminished. There will be times throughout the dying process when you will experience no fear at all, when peace and tranquillity will descend on you and life will be restored to a kind of balance. These periods will come and go. Remarkably, there will still be laughter and joy to be experienced, even after receiving such a terrifying diagnosis.

Grasping

After you've absorbed the shock and felt the fear, your mind will probably create a period of denial, in which you clutch at the idea of indefinite survival. Grasping is an outward expression of the fear you feel as you consider the fact that you are dying. Although many people fear leaving the world they know and the bodies they have inhabited, in my experience their greatest fear at this point is the fear of annihilation, of ceasing to exist as an entity in the universe. So they cling to the hope that somehow they can hang on permanently to this life.

For a brief time this can be a useful coping mechanism, but if you don't move beyond it, grasping can become a form of denial that persists throughout the dying process, preventing you from dealing with some of the essential emotional, psychological, and spiritual issues that confront you. Just as in any stage of life, your mind can focus on repetitive negative thoughts, leading to sadness and a paralysis of your will. (In Chapter 4, Step C, I will go into a more detailed look at the mind and how the awareness of its passions can help you overcome this potential difficulty.) The desire to cling to life can induce you to accept all kinds of treatments that have little or no therapeutic value, but only increase suffering. It's absolutely vital that you discern the difference between a treatment that has some real value and an approach that, even if it prolongs your life temporarily, significantly diminishes the quality of your remaining time. If you can do this, you have a valuable tool for making your choices. Perhaps a few more days or weeks of life are worth the extra suffering. Or perhaps a better quality of life is more important than a little extra time. Grasping for improbable cures is often fueled by the strong desire to get more time in this life. When faced with the reality of an end-of-life disease, some people increase their grasping for material objects in pursuit of pure pleasure. Like all the emotional reactions we'll be looking at, grasping can to some extent be healthy, and some degree of it will probably exist in everyone.

Your hope for survival can manifest itself with a desire to fight advancing disease and accept the awaiting hardships involved in uncomfortable treatments. This isn't completely bad. People clinging to life can often accomplish near miracles, especially when they have a specific event to live for. We've all heard stories of people who have lived far beyond their prognosis in order to witness a child's wedding or a grandchild's birth. And, of course, there are a handful of people who, told by their doctors they'd live for a year, lived for twenty. I would never discourage anyone from holding onto hope for as long as it seems reasonable. A healthy balance between hope and reality usually produces an understanding and acceptance of unfolding events. But at some point, you'll want to accept the inevitable: the time for miracles will have passed.

A seventy-year-old former executive I worked with who had metastatic colon cancer focused only on his desire to beat the odds and live to one hundred. Listening carefully to Mr. Sherman, I realized that his fear and denial of his end-of-life disease caused him to grasp for endless time in this life. Everything he said and did focused on this one goal—to buy more time. He made all his personal and medical decisions on this basis. He refused to grieve for his losses and face the future—the real future. He died without ever giving himself and his loved ones the opportunity to work through the issues of his life or his dying.

In contrast, Mr. Fillipio, also age seventy, who had advanced lung cancer, stayed briefly in denial after the diagnosis but soon began to talk to me about his impending death. "I still hope I'll live for years," he told me, "but I don't think that's going to happen." He asked me about other patients I'd worked with, and how they moved past wanting to live forever and accepted the realities of dying. We talked about ways of letting go of fear and grasping, even for a few moments, and Mr. Fillipio discovered his own way of coming to peace with his dying. He spent a lot of time with his family and focused on his love of poetry and music. Within a few weeks, he gave me a poem he had written expressing his hope for more quality days of living and a prayer for his wife to be able to accept his death.

Grief

When you have begun to accept the dying process, you have entered the grieving stage. You grieve for the imminent loss of your life as you know it. You grieve over lost opportunities, mistakes you can't undo, all the "roads not taken." At this point you begin the work of healing old wounds—your own as well as those of others. Memories of the mistakes you made that hurt others often emerge now, and you may experience a need to be forgiven for things you have done to others. You'll look back at your life, considering the pain you've caused people. Many people realize, consciously or unconsciously, that they've hurt loved ones. For some, the hurts have been great; for others, much less so. But since most humans make mistakes, nearly everyone has something to regret, and most people need to know that their loved ones can still see the good in their lives.

Grief emerges for many people during the dying process in such stark relief because they see as never before how important love, forgiveness, and gentleness are in life. It's healthy to experience grief at this stage. If you feel remorse for past actions and want to express that remorse to the people involved, it's a good idea to do so. Ask forgiveness. In turn, forgive those who have hurt you. And give your love.

But be prepared for a range of responses. The people you express your feelings to may not be ready to respond in kind. But it's still likely that your efforts will touch them deeply and, with time, help transform their feelings about themselves and you. By expressing your grief and remorse, by asking to be forgiven and by forgiving, you help heal others and bring peace to your own heart at this most important time of your life.

You may want to take comfort from a clergy member. Do not hesitate to ask your nurse, doctor, or family to ask one to visit you. You also might want to talk to a counselor or therapist;

again, act on this desire. Reach out to friends, family, and helping professionals—to anyone you can share your deepest feelings with, or derive the most comfort from. Both grief and the dying process are isolating, and both bring with them a yearning to reach out and feel united with other people, especially those you love.

One of my patients, Mr. Trattoria, had been angry and violent with his family, especially with his four children, throughout much of his life. At ninety-three he suffered from severe heart disease. His doctors offered him the small possibility that surgery might bring about recovery, though they said that, given his condition, the operation was risky and might not be successful even if he survived it. He was ambivalent, but at his wife's urging, he underwent the operation. Although Mr. Trattoria survived the surgery, he emerged from the operating room even closer to death. It was now clear that there would be no more surgeries or treatments. Barring divine intervention, Mr. Trattoria had only a short time to live. Yet he made the most of that time, because he responded to his grief and to the needs that it awakened in him.

He turned to the members of his family and begged their forgiveness for his abusive behavior over the years. He told each of them how much he loved them and how frightened he had always been of life. As he said to me just before he died, "I was so hard on my children that I ruined my family. I said to each of them, 'I am sorry. My anger came from my fear. I always believed that if I didn't do things just right, my life would be ruined. I had too much pride. I was arrogant. I wanted everyone to reflect well on me. If you didn't behave just as I wanted. . . .' " He made a slapping gesture.

Miraculously, Mr. Trattoria's honesty and love, which had finally emerged, brought forth forgiveness from his children and wife. He could not make the past right, but his honesty about his behavior, combined with the fact that he was dying, somehow reduced his children's need to express their anger to him. I remember how that family huddled around him at the end, knowing that he was dying, but drawing closer to one another, as if clinging to the life they shared and the love they felt for each other.

By accepting his own imminent death, Mr. Trattoria made his remaining days a time of forgiveness, letting go, and healing. Only by accepting death could he realize that it was time to experience and express his grief and remorse.

Of course, some people genuinely feel very little grief or remorse, because they've lived their lives with integrity and compassion. They may have a few regrets, but by and large they remain comfortable with who they've been and how they've treated others. And some have no regrets because, though they know they've done damage to others, they remain cold and remorseless. Those who have lived compassionately tend to move on to letting go, healing, and serenity very easily, often helped by family and friends who surround them. Those who reject any feelings of remorse tend to remain in fear or grasping until the very end, often leaving life with bitterness.

Letting Go

Eventually you'll begin the process of letting go: you begin to accept that the transition is under way. As you're dying, your mind struggles valiantly to survive, refusing to accept that your body is about to die. At this point, body and mind are in conflict. You are still in the grasping phase of the process. Accepting that you're dying is an act of letting go of the physical body and the identity that you associate with the body and your life. (In Chapter 4, the section on relaxation and meditation on pages 58 through 63 provides ways of working with the mind to help a person let go.)

If you believe in an existence after this life, letting go is a pivotal moment in the dying process during which you shift from existing as a physical being to existing as a spiritual being. You no longer identify exclusively with your body. Indeed, you begin to look forward to the life beyond. You gaze directly into your vision of the next world and embrace the mystery that is about to be opened up to you.

Many people are able to see their lives from an entirely new perspective at this stage, and consequently the meaning of their lives emerges as never before. They like to talk about what it meant for them to live, what they accomplished, what they learned. At this stage, you may come to realize what the purpose of your life was and how you fulfilled that purpose. As one of my patients said, "Life is a schoolhouse. You come here to learn certain lessons. Once you learn your lessons, you move on to another level of learning."

Whether or not you share such beliefs, letting go is a crucial stage. People who grasp for every extra moment, even through their final days of life, fill those days with fear and despair rather than with a peaceful resignation.

Mr. Edmunds, a sixty-year-old man I worked with, had fought kidney disease complicated by heart and lung failure for many years. He had been hospitalized in the intensive care unit more than eight times, and had been on dialysis for six years. Now advanced heart disease was causing him to be short of breath most of the time, and he was unable to get out of bed.

One day while I was sitting at his bedside, he looked up and said to me, "You know, Doc, I've been fighting this body of mine for over twelve years—and I plan to keep fighting as hard as I can." He looked over at all the get-well cards behind him—testimony to his loved ones' difficulty in accepting that this hospitalization would probably be his last. "But let me tell you," he added, "I've learned to keep fighting to stay alive without worrying about it. What will be will be. I'm afraid of death, but it's going to happen sometime."

Healing

The healing stage of the dying process occurs when you are able to see life's lessons, forgive yourself, and accept your life without judgment. Forgiveness is almost always accompanied by the realization that your life has had meaning, that your experiences have been purposeful, and that you have learned a great deal from being alive. Once you forgive yourself and realize that you have benefited from life, you are able to enter ever more deeply into compassion and self-love. You are also able to extend such feelings to others. When healing occurs at this level, it transcends all bitterness, regret, and self-condemnation.

One of my patients had lived his life on the periphery of society, taking odd jobs here and there. After regular brushes with the law, Gary had wound up in prison for several years for stealing a car. Only in his early fifties, Gary suffered from advanced and inoperable liver cancer. He came to spend the last months of his life at the Veteran's Administration Hospital in upstate New York, where I was a consulting hospice physician.

"What do you think is going to happen to me when I get to the other side?" he asked me one day while I sat with him in his room. "Do you think I'm going to have to deal with an angry God? Do you think people get punished? I'm scared of hell, to tell you the truth."

I told him that I felt strongly that he would not have to face an angry God.

"Yeah, but I've done a bunch of bad things," he said.

"Can you envision someone having enough love for you to understand everything and forgive you? I think the place we're all going is a hundred times more loving and understanding than anything we can imagine."

"A lot of what I've done came out of my own anger and self-hatred. I guess I'm afraid of being punished by a God that's also angry and full of hatred for me," he said.

For the next few weeks, I encouraged Gary to tell his life story, both by writing down his recollections and by talking about them to me and the people in his hospice ward. I also asked him to keep meditating on a loving, understanding, and forgiving universe. He did all of this, reflecting on his past as thoroughly as anyone I have ever worked with. In many of our sessions he told me about choices he had made that he now considered mistakes. Gary shed a lot of tears during his last few weeks of life.

Changes occur in people at the time of death that do not seem possible during ordinary life, when death seems remote. In the last weeks of his life, Gary underwent a remarkable transformation. As he became more introspective, his attitude became lighter and softer, especially toward himself. The angry scowl that had seemed molded into his face softened into a gentle, open countenance.

Just before Gary died, we talked again about what he expected to find on the other side of physical existence. "I think I'm going to be all right," he said. "I don't think it's going to be bad."

Serenity

The kind of peace that Gary found is the final gift of dying, serenity. You will have completed all that you need to do for yourself, your family, and the other people in your life. Such a feeling makes it possible to embark on a new journey. The struggle is over. Your work here is almost complete. You are ready to die peacefully.

When this happens, your friends and family can feel the peace that you have achieved and are radiating. It is a final gift to yourself and to those you care about. Flowing from that serenity is a powerful message that you are fine, that all is well.

One patient who achieved such serenity was Mrs. Hodges, who, at eighty-five, was hospitalized for advanced colon cancer and a stroke, which had caused her to have difficulty speaking. Aware of her rapid deterioration, she confided in me, via writing, that she wanted to help her two sons be at peace with her dying. She was ready to leave this life, she said, but her children couldn't understand her decision to forgo any further medical tests or treatments.

We had several family meetings (see Chapter 5, Step F, and Chapter 10, Step Y). Mrs. Hodges was able to convince her sons that she was truly contented and ready to die. "I will be fine," she wrote on her yellow pad. "I am not afraid any more of dying, and I will always be with you." Her serenity helped not only her, but her beloved sons as well, accept the reality of death.

Invariably, the people who witness this stage are comforted and reassured. They share that comfort with one another. The words your loved ones and friends tell each other seem like clichés only because no words can capture the solace and sense of completion that you communicate to those who witness your death.

This entire book is a preparation for that moment when peace and serenity descend on you and on those you hold dear.

PART TWO

The Steps of FairCare:
Positive Living,
Peaceful Dying

CHAPTER 3

Individuality of Disease, Individuality of Choice

❧ STEP A ❧
Recognizing Individuality of Disease, Individuality of Choice

*T*HE PROCESS of peaceful dying begins with your decision to take responsibility for your care and for how the rest of your life will play out. You can start to master your fears and your sense of powerlessness by insisting that all important decisions governing the rest of your life be made by you. Everyone dies, but *your* dying process is unique to you. You have your own physical, psychological, and spiritual needs. Only you can determine what will provide you with peace of mind now. You not only have that right, but you must also take responsibility for creating the events of your dying.

Your first step in making your decisions is to obtain medical information about your condition. Once you have that, you can consider the various treatment options and ask your doctor what the possible and probable outcomes of such treatments are. With that information, you can decide which treatments to use.

But this isn't a one-time-only decision. You'll want to monitor yourself continually to determine whether the treatment is succeeding in its purpose and whether it is enhancing the quality of your life. If the treatment isn't meeting your expectations, you'll want to review other options. Many people I've worked with have chosen aggressive medical care when they were first diagnosed with an end-of-life disease. Typically, they have continued with such care as long as it has seemed to be giving them a longer life span and allowing them to live their lives as they wish. But, it usually becomes clear at some point that such treatment has done all it can for them and is only interfering with the quality of their remaining life. Some of them have stopped aggressive treatment, then decided later to resume it for a time; others have stopped once and never gone back to it.

When facing an end-of-life diagnosis, most people choose a plan aimed at curing the disease. For many, this survival-based choice makes sense, even when there is only a slim chance of survival. I worked with a gynecologist who was diagnosed with advanced metastatic breast cancer a year after the birth of her second child. The average survival rate with such a diagnosis is six to nine months, and only 10 percent of patients live another ten years. After talking with her husband, Dr. Flax decided to undergo a very aggressive treatment of chemotherapy and radiation. Above all, she wanted to spend as much time raising her children as possible. Some of her relatives advised her to spare herself the suffering of the treatments, since her chances of survival were so slight. But she stuck with her decision, and six months after the treatments went into remission. We can't say she was cured—this was only a few years ago, and we don't know how long the remission will last—but she made the decision that was clearly right for her at that time.

Other patients make different choices. John Paul, a sixty-two-year-old man, came to the hospice/palliative-care unit of the hospital where I work after deciding to stop his dialysis treatments. He had been fighting both kidney disease and heart disease for years; he now had diabetes and poor circulation, as a result of which his leg had been amputated and he had lost much of the vision in both eyes. He understood that stopping dialysis would kill him within ten days.

———————

When I first visited him, he was sitting up in bed. I sat on the chair beside him, introduced myself, and said, as I usually do, "Well, here we are." I paused, because we both knew that what I really meant was, "Here we are at the end of your life." But did he want to discuss that with me? I waited in silence.

John was very willing to talk about dying. "I've fought this stuff for sixteen years, and I've gone through a lot of pain," he told me. "But there's no quality to my life anymore. I don't need to prolong it with this machine." He didn't seem despondent, only realistic. We talked a lot about death and dying and worked through many of the twenty-six steps together. He died as he wanted to, peacefully and without regret.

You Decide

While you'll want to discuss all the possibilities with your doctor as well as with your family and friends, it's important that *you* be the one to make the actual decisions. Never simply turn these decisions over to your doctor. Doctors are trained to apply a standardized form of medicine to every disease state—there are protocols for advanced cancer, advanced AIDS, and advanced organ failure, among others. But you're not just a generic case of cancer or heart disease: you're an individual with a disease that manifests in a particular way with you and that has particular meaning to you.

I've had many patients with the same disease category, but I've never had two patients with precisely the same disease. One lung-cancer patient may want aggressive treatment; one may want less aggressive treatment or an alternative treatment like acupuncture or herbal remedies. One may want to live until his grandchild's wedding day; another may have no particular goal except to live as comfortably as possible until she dies. One may be most terrified of death itself, another of pain, another of losing control over bodily functions. People have different tolerances for pain, different fears, different hopes, different diseases. Diseases are the same only in medical charts, never in individuals' experiences.

Yet few doctors are trained to approach patients with an awareness of this complexity. Medical school teaches standard approaches to each disease. The only way to ensure that you will get the individual attention that allows you to develop a treatment choice appropriate to your particular needs is to get all the information yourself and then decide what is right for you; it is not to accept what your doctor believes is right for everyone in your circumstances.

If you decide that your doctor's advice isn't right for you, don't go along with it. My father-in-law, a seventy-year-old retired executive who was used to being in control of his life, struggled for some time with treatments for his metastatic esophageal cancer. He consulted with a leading oncologist at one of New York City's prestigious cancer specialty hospitals. The oncologist advised him to follow a very aggressive chemotherapy-radiation course, which gave him a small chance of surviving another six to nine months. My father-in-law decided instead to be treated by a homeopathic physician and to use classical homeopathic remedies. The young doctor at the cancer center was miffed. "If you don't undergo the treatments, you'll definitely die," he said.

"Young man," my father-in-law replied, "with all due respect, I have advanced metastatic cancer, and I'm seventy years old. I'll definitely die whether I accept your treatments or not. I'd prefer to die without side effects from radiation and chemotherapy." He left and worked with the alternative doctor, who was able to help make his dying comfortable. He died at home, in peace, his pain controlled; he was surrounded by his family and was helped by members of a local hospice group. It's not that the oncologist's advice was wrong, but that it was wrong for this particular man. Someone else might have jumped at even a tiny chance of a longer survival time.

View your doctor as one source of information—an important source—but not as the person who ultimately decides what course should be taken. Your doctor and hospital staff are experts hired by you to perform certain services—to work with you, not to dictate what you must do. You should certainly respect their expertise (if you don't, you want to look for replacements), but that's a lot different from treating them like gods.

This tendency to turn doctors into gods has a number of dangerous consequences. If doctors are gods, they can grant immortality. When they fail, as they must, people feel angry and disillusioned. This isn't only the doctors' fault. Western culture buys into this belief. Often we turn our responsibilities for ourselves over to the doctor-god.

It's also important not to surrender your decisions to family members. Those who love you may find it difficult to accept that you are dying, and wishful thinking can cause them to interpret your physical weakness as a sign that they must make your decisions for you. Although this is understandable, it is also unacceptable. You must make your family members understand that ultimately this is your death and you have the exclusive right to determine how your dying process should unfold. Their role is to help you look calmly at all the options available and at the same time help you recognize your responsibility in making critical choices for treatment. The only exception comes when you have legally turned over such decision making and appointed another person as your medical proxy. (A detailed explanation of the importance of securing a medical proxy and why advance directives and living wills are often ignored is presented in Chapter 6.)

I cannot emphasize enough how important it is for family

members to accept your decision. I've seen the devastating results of the failure to do this. When I was a medical intern, I worked at a large hospital as a house officer in charge of the intensive care and coronary care units for six consecutive weeks, working alternate twenty-four-hour shifts of one full day on, one day off, the next day on again, and so forth. On my twenty-fifth consecutive alternate day, a ninety-two-year-old woman was admitted for heart failure. Mrs. Rogers came into the hospital unconscious, curled up in the fetal position, her breathing shallow and labored.

On her chart were her advance directives, in which she clearly stated that no attempts should be made to resuscitate her and that she was to undergo absolutely no life-prolonging techniques in the face of irreversible disease.

By her hospital bedside were her two daughters, upset and anxious. Next to them, apparently much calmer, was Mrs. Rogers's granddaughter, a nurse at a local teaching hospital. Exhausted after too many nights in the coronary care unit, and assuming that I had a professional ally I could talk frankly with about the patient's advance directives, I asked the young woman what she thought of her grandmother's condition.

Suddenly, her expression changed. "We want to do everything for Grandma, everything possible!" she said passionately.

Caught completely off guard by her sudden release of emotion, I said, "Well, why don't we try a few medications to help her heart failure? But you know what 'everything' means, don't you? I assume you don't really want us to resuscitate your grandmother?" She knew as well as I did how aggressive a procedure this was.

The young nurse turned on me angrily. She insisted that *everything*, everything possible must be done to save her grandmother. How dare I suggest that we provide anything less than that?

Tired, angry, and feeling bound to defend the grandmother's written wishes, I asked the nurse if she knew of her grandmother's advance directives, which she was clearly violating. She simply repeated her demands that everything be done to keep Mrs. Rogers alive.

Finally I said, "If you really love your grandmother, you'll take her home and let her die in peace." Then I walked out of the room and asked my senior resident to take over the care of this patient. He agreed.

Mrs. Rogers was admitted to the coronary care unit and medicated. There she suffered another heart attack. I was called to her bedside for a code blue. I watched as a resident physician compressed the patient's tiny chest while a ventilation tube was placed down her throat. Her chest heaved up and down as the ventilator breathed for her mechanically. She remained attached to the breathing machine for several days, her dazed eyes wide open, staring out into the intensive care unit. Four days after admission, she developed pneumonia, and three days after that her heart stopped again. Another resuscitation was attempted to restart her heart; when this one failed, everyone left the room dejected.

I was responsible for pronouncing the patient, which meant calling the family to inform them of her death and then filling out the death certificate, the eighth one I had completed that day. As I entered the information on the forms, I thought about this woman, her explicit request not to be resuscitated, and how we had failed her.

The granddaughter's failure came from the fact that her feelings for her grandmother were too attached to her own needs. She had no doubt convinced herself that she was acting out of love, but in fact her actions showed that she did not care enough for her grandmother to respect her wishes. The hospital's failure came from its concept of professionalism, which was far too narrow in its vision of the healer's job.

Family members often have great difficulty in situations like this. They feel responsible for keeping the dying person alive. Even when someone has clearly asked to be allowed to die peacefully, I've often heard people say, "How can we just let him die? We have to do everything for him."

Sometimes this response comes less from love than from guilt. I see it a lot with people who have ignored their family for years and suddenly become reinvolved when one relative is dying. It's as though they're trying to overcompensate for their neglect by fighting to save the person's life. Instead, they compound whatever harm they did in the past by forcing their will on the dying person.

It's crucial, then, while you're still able to communicate, to make your family members understand that they must do everything to facilitate *your* wishes, whatever their own may be, that this is the demand you are making on their love. (I discuss talking to your family in more detail in Chapter 5, Step F.)

No one but you—not your family, not your doctor, not your counselor—can make this choice for you. Even this book should be only one other source of information to help guide you in your decision making. You can use each source selectively, choosing to accept certain recommendations or therapies while rejecting others.

Although there is a great deal for you to do now, there is still enough time in which to do it. Many people live a year, two years, or longer with a disease that will eventually end their lives. You may be confined to a bed for only a part of your dying process. There is time to reflect on life and to take up unresolved issues that you have postponed or avoided. You can accomplish a lot during this period, if you accept it for what it is. Only by establishing control and never relinquishing it can you be assured that you will experience peaceful dying.

CHAPTER 4

Taking Control of Your Life

❖ STEP B ❖
Confronting, Expressing, and Diminishing
Fear of Dying

WHILE YOU, the dying patient, are trying to deal with your fears, your family and even your doctors are experiencing fears of their own. All these fears—yours, those of your loved ones, and those of the medical staff—are affecting you. The worst effect of fear is that it can prevent you from being able to evaluate, contemplate, and plan your life. In addition, fear can prevent you from experiencing love, love for yourself and for those who have been important to you.

You need to deal with your fears to be able to fully appreciate the crises and opportunities that exist for you now. The most essential part of your work now is to do all you can to make love triumph over anxiety. It is tremendously important that you face your fear and the anger, pain, and frustration that go with it. We live in a culture that tries to anesthetize any emotional pain. We have a standardized image of how to feel and how to look. It's essentially a marketing image, an image of someone who looks perfect and is never hassled. It's an image that suggests that any problem can be solved by the right deodorant, peanut butter, or car.

But life is never that simple. Rather than anesthetize every discomfort, it makes sense to face the fear and confusion, feel it, and work through it. When you're in an end-of-life situation, it's important to drop as many masks as possible and to be with your feelings.

All the fears you now experience are a little different from one another. Initially, you feel shock and terror. It may take a while to be able to look at these emotions and work with them. Many people are paralyzed by fear in the beginning. This is perfectly natural. Western culture offers little guidance in confronting and diminishing the core denial of death we all experience. In some Eastern beliefs, such as Tibetan Buddhism, people meditate on their dying as part of a daily ritual, and fear of dying is not as great as it is in the West. Although Christian-based Western cultures include the concept of eternal existence, many people have not integrated this concept into their minds in a way that lessens their fear of dying.

You'll need time to deal with your own fears about dying, and you'll probably need help from others, both professionals and your own loved ones. However, in my experience, just recognizing how potent a force your fear of dying is will help you develop ways of confronting that fear. Once you've confronted it, you can work toward diminishing it. Instead of pushing the fear away, try to hold it for even a few seconds at a time and realize that you can and will work with this potentially overwhelming emotion.

Much of the fear of dying concerns the loss of your physical body. You ask yourself questions such as, Does this loss mean that I will no longer exist at all? If I do continue to exist, what form will I have once I let go of my body? Will I have consciousness? Will I be dispersed into the cosmic void, my molecules and consciousness scattered across space?

This question of an existence after death is one that patients often bring up with me. Most of them find comfort in the possibility of eternal existence and in the fact that virtually all religions include a belief in the eternal nature of soul.

If you are open to this idea, you may find it helpful, as have many of my patients, to do a little meditation about it. Begin with one of the breathing exercises described later in Step C. Then focus your attention on the possibility of eternal existence. See if the concept feels right to you. Many people find their fear of dying reduced dramatically when they experience the possibility of existing beyond their current life.

You will likely fear the loss of your identity and all that surrounds and supports that identity, including your personality, professional accomplishments, and material possessions. All that you have built in your life will apparently be gone. You wonder what, if anything, will take its place.

You will fear the loss of those you love—your spouse, lover, children, friends. How will they all fare without me? you ask. Who will protect, care for, and watch over my kids? Will my spouse find someone else? Do I *want* my spouse to find someone else? Will everyone forget me?

You will also fear the experience of pain, of losing bodily control, and of being confined to a bed. Will my pain become unbearable? you ask yourself. You will fear the shame and the sense of powerlessness: Will I become incontinent and be put into diapers? What will my life be like when I can't walk or get out of bed? Will they ever tie me into a chair or bed?

Sometimes the fear will come out as anger. I've seen many situations in which both patient and family have lashed out furiously at the doctors, the nurses, the hospital food—anything they could latch onto. Anger is usually more successful at masking pain than fear is, so fear gets wrapped in anger. You can even become angry at yourself, thinking, If I hadn't smoked so much or drunk so much or eaten so much fatty food, none of this would have happened. Logically these issues no longer matter, and you don't want to get stuck in your anger. But it's important to feel it, let it out, and see what it really means. Most of all, be gentle with yourself. You must realize that there are ways to deal with the fear, anger, and other feelings that will arise at times, often with great intensity.

Facing and discussing your fears can lessen their power over you, pulling them into the light instead of leaving them buried in your unconscious, where they can control the decisions you make without your even realizing it. Furthermore, failure to express your fears can prevent you from getting the help you need and keep you in a state of numbness and isolation. This entire book, including each of the steps, is directed toward giving you the language to deal with your fear and denial of death. These fears can lead you to answers and eventually to peace.

It might help to make a list of all your fears and then discuss each fear with the appropriate person—a member of the clergy, a counselor, your spouse, one of your children, a friend, a business partner, even your health care worker. Too often valuable conversation between the health care worker and the dying person is lost because the health care worker fails to ask the simple question, "What are your fears about the days and months ahead?"

Mr. Murray, a forty-eight-year-old patient I counseled, was confined to his bed with end-stage AIDS. He saw that the medical team visiting him on rounds one morning looked uncomfortable, so he smiled and jokingly said, "Now I know what it feels like to be a monkey in the zoo. Stop staring at me and say something nice!"

His attending physician smiled thinly and began to talk about medical facts. Finally Mr. Murray broke in. "Listen, guys," he said. "You all seem more unhappy about my dying than I am! I've fought this disease for years, and I'm scared of dying—but not *that* scared!" He grinned broadly and then said, more soberly, "Look, what I need is people I can talk with about my fears—not to pretend they don't exist." The entire team was impressed by his forthrightness and began to help him talk over his fears about what his dying would be like.

Only by facing your fears can you let growth and healing occur. I've seen this over and over with my patients. Sometimes they are quiet in their denials. Other times, they're very blunt— like Mrs. Shapiro, an elderly patient with advanced kidney and lung disease. I had thought she was fairly at peace with dying. She was constantly smoking, which was surely hastening her inevitable death. But when I first suggested that she and her family might want to think about preparing for her death, she was furious. "Don't even mention that word!" she snapped.

When I tried to probe further, she said that she would not entertain the thought that she was dying. "I refuse to think about it," she told me, and turned away.

Mrs. Shapiro was unusual only in her bluntness. Like most of us, she had spent her life denying death; she was not about to change now. She never faced her emotions about dying, even when she entered the hospital for the last time, her kidneys beginning to close down. She refused any counseling and insisted that she be left alone. Her dying in isolation appeared emotionally painful. Her facial expressions showed fear, and she was constantly tense; she appeared incapable of even a moment of complete relaxation.

Fortunately, Western culture is beginning to change this determination to ignore the inevitable. There are a number of reasons for this change. The baby boomers are aging, facing their parents' deaths and their own mortality. Many of the new spirituality movements, as well as revivals in traditional religions, are causing people to question the nature of death and their own beliefs about the soul. The debate about assisted suicide has spawned public discussion of pain management and end-of-life care.

Everyone needs help and guidance in moving through the specific fears of dying. My experience with the dying has led me to believe that there is a mysterious process at hand that is awakening people at this stage to other dimensions of their lives, which makes possible the ability to move into a time of contemplating dying and whatever may come after it.

I have seen extraordinary examples of how facing fears head-on can free people and help create peaceful deaths. Shortly after I began my work as a palliative physician in the hospice ward of a VA hospital, a sixty-eight-year-old man with advanced pancreatic cancer was admitted. His attending physician, a nurse practitioner, a staff psychologist, and I went to see him to answer any questions he might have. But Mr. Williams had only one question, and it was for his internist.

"Are there any more treatments that could help me?" he asked.

"No, sir," the doctor answered. "I don't think treatment of any kind can cure your cancer."

Mr. Williams began to cry, but quickly cut his tears short and regained his composure.

"I'm sorry," he said. "I used to be called the Destroyer Man. I would never cry; that was my standard."

I leaned over to him and said that people in the last stage of life have a chance, if they choose it, to change some of their lifelong standards.

The next day I visited Mr. Williams and asked how he was doing. He nodded and looked down at the floor. "I'm fine, doing just fine," he said. He was very polite—and very stoic.

I went to see him regularly after that in the hope that he might open up, but each time he walled himself off from me. Finally on one of my visits, his cold exterior melted and he confessed that he was terrified of dying. He could not bear the thought of leaving his wife, who had Alzheimer's disease, and his two grown children. He had many financial concerns that he felt would burden his family. Finally, and quite sheepishly, Mr. Williams confided that he was afraid of having to pay for many of the actions taken in this life when he passed on to the next.

Expressing these fears was a breakthrough for this man. He had spent his entire life being strong for himself and others, erecting barriers against fears that he considered shameful. Gathering his courage now, he took a great step into the unknown, and in the process moved from the grasping stage to grieving and letting go.

I did not advise Mr. Williams at all when he first began talking, but simply gave him the opportunity to talk about his fears and to confess his pain and regrets. Over several meetings that followed, I would sit by his bedside and simply listen to him, hearing his statements without judging him. My only desire was to communicate that I respected him and enjoyed his company, which I sensed was what he wanted from me. As his dying progressed, Mr. Williams began to talk to me about the moment when he, like many before him, would take in his last breath, breathe out, and peacefully let it go. He considered this for a long time. He had many questions about other deaths I had witnessed, and I was happy to share some of my relevant experiences.

"Will I experience a lot of pain?" Mr. Williams asked.

"No. We have very effective pain medication," I assured him. "All you have to do is allow us to help you by telling us how much pain you are in." His pain was being managed expertly by the staff at the VA hospital; he would be comfortable throughout the remaining months of his life.

The mere act of confronting the things Mr. Williams was most afraid of began to reduce his fears. It also changed his demeanor dramatically. He began to look forward to my arrival, he told me. He cried regularly, releasing a lifetime of unshed tears. Crying was cathartic now. Gradually, his manner and spirit lightened. Despite his concerns, he laughed frequently. Both of us knew that this laughter was a powerful tool for confronting and lessening his worry.

Dealing with his fears also allowed him to open up to his two children, to whom he confided his concerns about his wife and their future, and he felt better. At my suggestion, the three of them set up a series of meetings at which they could address their practical and financial concerns. Following those meetings, they also discussed many long-standing family issues. Both of his children had painful memories and anger that they wanted to share with their father. Mr. Williams had much to say to them as well. A great deal of pain had been stored up inside him, but he had longed for the opportunity to say he was sorry for many of his actions and also to explain his motivations. He told his children how difficult his life had been and how much he wanted to provide the best he could for them and his wife. He had made many mistakes, but he had also tried his best. As he told me later, these discussions with his children gave him an experience of redemption and peace he could never have envisioned.

Addressing fears of dying and long-repressed emotions is a significant turning point in the dying process, because it allows you to proceed from the early phases of fear and grasping toward healing and serenity, which Mr. Williams achieved. Both he and his family were comforted and very much at peace when he took in and released his last breath. He had completed his journey.

Your Family's and Friends' Fears

Knowing you have family and friends who love you can be of enormous comfort when you are dying. But it can also cause stress. You'll need to deal not only with your own fears, but with theirs as well. Dealing with your mortality forces them to face their own fears of dying. They may project these fears onto you. People you have always relied on may suddenly distance themselves from you. Others may speak to you in pitying or patronizing ways, just when you most need them to be fully honest with you.

You need to recognize that these fears are natural. Your loved ones are facing not only a terrible loss, from which they may feel a need to protect themselves, but their own mortality as well.

When these loved ones are your children, even if they are self-sufficient adults, they still have some sense of being abandoned, even orphaned. The impending loss of parents can trigger deep, survival-based emotions that are strong and somewhat complex. Parents have an aura of immortality. They were there when the child came into the world. The fact that they can leave that world may terrify even the most mature and balanced adult child.

Spouses, lovers, and close friends are also facing a terrible loss. All your loved ones may be unconsciously and irrationally angry with you, both for leaving them and for being a reminder that they too will one day die.

They may also fear that they will never be able to reconcile long-standing issues with you, that old wounds will remain forever open. They may want to say things to you but fear that doing so will contribute to your suffering. You should encourage them not to hold back. This may help enable them to say what they need to in a gentle and loving way without compromising what they feel. Often people are afraid their emotions are too strong, and they can be paralyzed by their fear of hurting you. In that case, they should talk to family members, close friends, a psychologist, or a grief counselor. (Such assistance is explained in Chapter 5, Steps E, F, and H.) It is just as important for your loved ones to confront and express fears as it is for you to do so.

At the same time, it's better if all of you can avoid hysteria and emotional outbursts. The purpose of this time is reconciliation and reunion: you need to be both honest and loving with each other. Sometimes these goals may seem at odds with each other, even between healthy people. Most of us at times conceal anger or disappointment from those we love in order to avoid hurting them. Try as best you can to be honest now, framing hurtful thoughts in kind and loving language. This is what creates peaceful dying. (These points are discussed in more detail in Chapter 5, Steps F and G.) In the process of becoming conscious of your fears and expressing them, you can all find comfort and support.

Sometimes the family's fears cause more suffering for the dying person than does dying itself. This is especially true with young children. I have seen again and again, as have many other doctors I know, that children are less fearful of dying than are adults. But for parents facing the unspeakable anguish of losing a child, this can be hard to understand.

One patient I worked with early in my training was a nine-year-old girl who had advanced leukemia. Melissa had gone through several years of chemotherapy and difficult hospitalizations. She had experienced many painful procedures.

Understandably, her parents were having a difficult time adjusting to her approaching death. But their emotions often got the best of them. Her father, angry and bitter, lashed out at the nurses. He and his wife bickered constantly in front of their child.

One day when I was examining her, Melissa told me she wanted to discuss something. "Doctor Dan," she said thoughtfully, "I know I'm dying. I'm going to be in heaven soon, with my dog, Blackie. I'm not afraid to go to heaven—it seems like that's what I have to do. But I wish my parents would stop hurting so much. I hate it when they're always fighting." Sadly, her parents' confusion and pain was so great that they couldn't alter their behavior, and they were unable to learn the lesson their wiser child had to teach them. Their actions upset Melissa more and more. Soon, whenever I came into the room, I would find her lying in bed with the sheets pulled over her head. Her parents' behavior had driven this open, courageous child into a somber retreat.

Your Doctors' Fears

Virtually all doctors have witnessed many deaths in their professional careers, yet few of them are able to accept or cope with death well. In struggling to keep patients alive, doctors are like soldiers fighting a war in which they can win only individual battles, never the whole conflict. In the end, everyone dies. Death in the case of a terminally ill patient is not a failure of medicine or of the individual doctor. It is a natural event that physicians are only now beginning to accept.

Doctors also have their own fear of death. Oddly enough, medical training rarely deals with this fear. But people who deal with the dying won't be effective unless they're able to confront the fact that they too are mortal and to face the terrors this knowledge can bring. Doctors all too often transfer their own unconscious fears onto their patients: each death they can't prevent is a reflection of the ultimate death they can't prevent—their own. They face their patients not with empathy—the concern that arises from a deep knowledge of human similarity—but with pity, a more distanced emotion.

Another fear that makes it difficult for doctors to do anything but treat the underlying disease, even when such treatment is obviously hopeless, is the fear of a malpractice suit. A doctor who does not use the "best available" (defined always as though that meant "most advanced" or "most dramatic") treatments faces the possibility of a lawsuit because decisions may be questioned later on by the family or by the local medical board. In many cases, doctors are required to conform to existing practices, even if they feel these practices are of questionable value.

You can help your doctor give you appropriate treatment and stop it when it becomes inappropriate by discussing all your desires in advance and by putting your wishes in an advance directive such as a living will (see Chapter 6, Step I). Finally, you can ensure that your desires are followed by carefully discussing them with your loved ones as well as by appointing a medical proxy.

✷ STEP C ✷
Slowing Down Time and the Mind

When you've been diagnosed with a life-threatening or end-stage disease, events seem to speed up and develop a momentum all their own. You can easily feel victimized by your circumstances, overcome with a sense of powerlessness. At this point, you must remember that dying can take weeks, months, and even years. During every moment left to you, there is life to be lived. You have many important things to accomplish, both for yourself and for those you care about.

An essential part of slowing down the events and reclaiming control is to follow the wise old adage: take one day and one decision at a time. As much as possible, remain in the present, the here and now. Take whatever comfort you can in this moment. You do not have to address anything that is not required today. As much as possible, look to the positive aspects of every situation. Positive thinking can allow better events to occur by creating the opportunity for your wishes to be fulfilled. Drowning in negative thoughts can paralyze you.

Most people decide to undergo some treatments aimed at curing their disease, or at least at prolonging their lives. This is perfectly reasonable. Treatments for cancer, AIDS, and a number of deadly diseases can extend life for longer periods of time than was possible in the past, and with their help you may live for quite a while longer. Once in a great while, such a treatment actually cures a supposedly "incurable" disease. It's important for you to learn all the possible side effects of any treatment you undertake so that you can cope with it as comfortably as possible. Even with the best of these treatments, your life will change a great deal, and you'll need to take all the changes into account. For instance, radiation and chemotherapy can weaken you, and you're likely to experience a decrease in your energy level and your ability to live your life as you used to.

With all the new experimental drugs reported in the news almost daily, you might want to try to become part of a protocol, an experimental group being treated by a new process to see whether it works. You're taking a gamble if you do—experiments usually don't work. But there are two possible advantages: if it works, you might be able to slow down the process of your disease for many years; if it doesn't work, you're participating in something that may give medical science knowledge that can help others in the future.

You must also realize that, at least initially, your range of emotions is going to be limited by your fears. You need to examine your fears and work with them. Many other feelings also exist within you that could help shape your experience if you allow them to surface. Are you acknowledging your own feelings of loss? A certain amount of grieving is inevitable at this stage. Holding in such feelings can lead to brooding, melancholy, and depression. Let them out and you will be supported by your underlying feelings of love, which, if you can connect with them, will strengthen your ability to face the future without so much fear and self-doubt.

Being receptive now means slowing down, awakening to all that you feel, and allowing yourself to be helped by those around you. I have seen connecting with feelings work wonders in many patients. One patient I worked with was a gruff professor of economics who had been diagnosed with metastatic and incurable stomach cancer. His wife tried to talk with him about his impending death, but he refused to discuss it with her or to make any plans for the months ahead.

We worked on this for a time, and eventually he was able to contemplate his life and talk with his family. At first, he didn't do anything; he simply allowed himself to think about the idea of improving communications with his family. When he was ready, he approached his family. Instead of holding in the issues he wanted to share and resolve, he took control of the situation. He apologized to his family for having been so caught up in his career that he had spent little time with them, and he asked to be forgiven. Now he understood that he had been crowding his mind with anger, denial, anything he could to avoid accepting his inevitable death. Letting go of all those thoughts and focusing on how he could best use the last months of his life led him to a peaceful, resolved dying, surrounded by the people he loved.

Relaxation and Meditation

As much as possible, spend time quieting your mind each day. Twenty minutes or more of silent relaxation, meditation, contemplation, or prayer can bring you tremendous comfort and peace, allowing you to be guided by the spiritual forces that surround and imbue your life. It can also help you evaluate your situation to determine whether you will proceed with a specific treatment, how you want to modify your advance directives (see Chapter 6, Step I), and how you want to deal with an array of practical concerns.

Many people like to combine prayer with meditation. Ask for the guidance you need, especially when you are confronted with important decisions. Find quiet spaces and time to be alone, but also share the insights and revelations that arise from these meditative states with those who love you.

You may need to experiment with various techniques in order to decide which will work for you. Relaxation techniques may be all you want or need, or you may want to use meditation techniques as well. Meditation is the practice of quieting the mind and allowing yourself to experience the light and sound within you. Meditation quiets the mind and emotions, allowing them to emerge clearly. It may be helpful to envision your mind, emotions, and soul as separate. (*The New World Dictionary of the American Language* defines *soul* as "an entity which is regarded as being the immortal or spiritual part of the person.")

Many techniques will slow down your experience of time and allow you to experience considerable control. I'm including a few techniques here. You may want to read about them all, or you may want to read only about those that interest you.

RELAXATION

Relaxation techniques are the simplest of the mind-quieting methods. The easiest technique is simply to sit in silence for eight to ten minutes. Choose a silent spot if one is available to you; if not, try to shut out any distractions around you. Catch any thought that enters your mind. Recognize that such thoughts aren't really silence, and let them go, trying to make your mind a blank. It may help to close your eyes and try to keep a blank screen in the area between your eyes at the middle of your fore-head.

Another very basic technique is to pay attention to your breathing. Sit quietly in a comfortable position and gently inhale (through your nose if possible) for a slow count of eight; then gently exhale through your mouth to the same count of eight. Do this five times and then stop. Begin again, this time without counting, but trying to keep the same approximate amount of time. Continue doing this for eight to twenty minutes. If you find thoughts entering your mind, especially stressful ones, just let them go and return your attention to your breathing. Don't be alarmed or dismayed if you find that thoughts keep returning: they will. Just keep letting them go. You should be able to sense yourself slowing down.

If you choose, you can stop here. Your brief silent time will have done you a lot of good. But you may wish to go further. Listen to your intuition. You may feel drawn to pray or meditate. If so, follow that feeling.

CHANTING

There are also some mind-body techniques you may find useful. One that I've found very helpful in my own life over the years uses the strengthening effect of sound. It consists of combining the breathing technique and the silent time just described with a chant or a single word or combination of words—what's known as a mantra. The traditional Eastern *om* is a mantra, but you may prefer something else. One sound that people often use is *hu* (rhymes with *you*). Some people prefer an actual word, such as *peace*. You can also use a brief phrase from a favorite prayer. Once you've chosen your chant, begin the technique.

First, inhale and then, as you exhale, speak your word or phrase. Repeat this for about eight to twenty minutes.

VISUALIZATION

You might want to add to your technique a visualization that many of my patients have found helpful. Imagine a large circle of blue or white light shining on the top of your head, directly over you. Transform that light into the feeling of pure love and mercy. Feel the entire universe pouring its warmth and love onto you through this circle of light.

If you have trouble feeling this light, think about someone you have loved deeply—a parent, spouse, child, friend, even a pet. Put that love into the circle of light that is showering down on you.

Try to allow that light and love to connect with your deepest self for at least a few moments. Imagine the light filling you, from your head down to your neck, your chest and arms, your stomach, your legs, your feet and your toes. Allow the light to comfort your worried mind and trust that it will help you in the days ahead to carry forward and do well with whatever you experience. Most of all, try to bask in the light and love without asking for anything specific.

If you wish, you can visualize a particular spiritual figure, perhaps one central to your religion, such as Jesus or Buddha. Alternatively, you might borrow a figure from a spiritual system you're drawn to but not part of. You do not need to visualize a traditional religious figure: any spiritual guide or guardian angel that resonates with you will work well.

Another visualization technique is to pretend you're a fly in the corner of the ceiling looking at you, and appreciate how hard you are working to reach a peaceful state. Visualize a shower of light spreading all over yourself, and experience the power of seeing meditation as a light-gathering experience.

AFFIRMATIONS

Another technique is that of affirmation. It's a variation on the idea of "whistling a happy tune." Say to yourself simple phrases expressing the state you wish to be in: "I am peaceful and contented"; "I am physically comfortable"; "I love and am loved by the universe." It's very important to phrase affirmations positively. If you say, "I do not feel pain," you're implanting the idea of pain in your mind. Sometimes using positive expressions can be difficult; it's hard to say, "I am peaceful and contented," when you're terrified. An alternative is to phrase your thought in terms of choice: "I choose to be peaceful and contented," or "I choose peace and tranquillity."

STICK WITH IT!

While you're meditating, experience and appreciate whatever comes to you. Building a meditative technique and practice, like all other important work, takes time and perseverance. Keep your mind free of thoughts as best you can. If you catch your first thought going to a routine worry or flight of ideas, catch the specific idea and hold onto it. Give the worry or fear a moment of recognition and try to see yourself in a loving manner, from above or from somewhere else in the room, worrying about the specific thought. Capturing this moment will often allow you to return to a meditative state with an appreciation of how your mind can race to other thoughts and distract you from peaceful meditation.

You can bring any of these techniques informally into your daily life. Just think, occasionally, of the endless special feelings and potential for embracing the light and sound of peace that you will often experience while meditating. You can try to give that peace and love to your friends, relatives, and others in tense daily situations. The ability to relate to a peaceful, loving feeling and to experience it in a difficult situation may become one of the many benefits of your meditative work. You can also use visualization at different times during the day—while you're showering or resting. A simple variant is to picture yourself pain free and fearless in the face of your impending death. You can also use the white-light visualizations described earlier at any time, not only during meditation. And you can *always* do affirmations; even if you have only ten seconds, you can say to yourself, "I choose to be peaceful."

WHEN IT DOESN'T WORK

Meditation and related techniques can be very helpful to most people. But for some people, they simply don't work. Although it's worth putting a little initial effort into making it work, don't keep pushing yourself if it doesn't. In *How to Meditate*, Lawrence LeShan offers some very sensible advice. A meditation program, he says, should always make you feel better when you do it than when you do not do it. He suggests that after each meditation, you compare the way you feel to how you felt before you began. If the work you are doing is the right kind of work for you, then most of the time the answer will be that you feel better, more "put together." If you don't, LeShan says, drop the meditation program and try another.* Finally, if you have a sense that meditation is wrong for you, don't do it.

Psychological Patterns

Another helpful tool in slowing down your mind is becoming aware of the psychological patterns that involve the effects of childhood trauma. These are powerful patterns that play out throughout your life and are particularly strong as your end-of-

---

* Lawrence LeShan, *How to Meditate* (New York: Bantam Books, 1974), pp. 33, 39.

life situation unfolds. Being aware of them can help you observe and control your mind.

For people who have had difficult childhoods, the scars often remain throughout life. I have been struck with how many of the patients I've worked with—even quite elderly ones—have talked about events in their childhood that filled them with deep feelings of loneliness, abandonment, helplessness, and shame. Often such feelings emerge as people deal with their present families.

Healing this childhood trauma is never easy work, and it may require years of psychotherapy—years that you may not have at this point. Moving forward from childhood events is easier for some people than for others. Still, being aware that some of your current patterns may be directly related to childhood incidents can be extremely helpful. Recognizing that old emotions may be directing some of your adult behavior and creating stressful patterns can help lessen the power of those patterns. When you find your own way of addressing the old pain, you can help resolve some of your current deep personal conflicts. You can begin forgiving the people in your past and seeing life in a more positive light.

If recognizing the wounds proves not to be enough, you can turn to one of the many forms of brief, short-term psychotherapy directed at examining two or three patterns that are causing discomfort. Cognitive therapy as well as other situational counseling may be helpful for such issues. You can ask your primary doctor for a referral to a qualified counselor or therapist who practices one of these forms.

In addition to childhood trauma, you can find yourself trapped in the passions of the mind. These passions can exist in anyone, and they range from mild to obsessive. If you develop an awareness of them, you can control them better. Greed, anger, vanity, extreme attachment, and lust are the major passions of the mind. The mnemonic *gavel* can help you remember these five passions and identify their presence. Once you can identify them, there's a chance to free yourself from them if you feel they are holding you back.

Greed. This excessive need for accumulating material objects starts from a very sensible desire to support yourself and your family, but it mushrooms into something with a life of its own. Although it provides great gratification in its early stages, when it grows, it can supplant any other criteria for self-worth. Think of the common colloquialism that defines someone with a certain amount of money as being worth that amount: "He's worth two million dollars." When you think of your worth in terms of your material possessions, you're trapped into a pattern of greed. This pattern can dull your sensibilities to the real needs of others, particularly of those with fewer possessions—who are "worth" less than you. It can also fuel resentment toward those who have more than you.

Most of all, greed can hinder your ability and willingness to look at other aspects of living and dying. Defining your human worth and letting go of actions that may represent greed will help you become peaceful with your living and your dying.

Anger. Anger as an immediate response is a healthy emotion. You hurt me; I'm angry at you. Holding on to anger after its moment has passed, however, causes emotional damage. Often it turns inward, resulting in physical ailments and depression. At the same time, it can turn outward, not only toward people who have hurt you, but toward those who haven't as well. This is why, for example, children who have been abused by their parents so often abuse their own children. It isn't accidental that another term for angry is *mad*—anger that isn't resolved can become a kind of insanity. Recognizing your old angers and trying to resolve them and let go of them can be tremendously healing at any time. It is particularly important as you are coming to the end of your life. If possible, forgive the people who have harmed you, recognizing that they too were probably acting out of old, unresolved angers. If you can't forgive them, at least try to let go of as much of your anger as possible.

Vanity. It's pleasant to enjoy the way you look, to dress and adorn yourself in attractive ways. But excessive focus on physical attractiveness causes you to identify yourself with your appearance. It would be dangerous enough if you simply felt you were extremely beautiful and valued that above your other qualities, but today in our culture much attention is focused on changing appearance—hiding wrinkles, coloring hair, dieting. This creates a view that your natural body is inadequate. Aging exacerbates these feelings, and the desire to live up to an image of perfection can become obsessive. When you reach an end-of-life situation, vanity can be devastating. Treatments may cause hair loss and other challenges to your physical self-image, and the dying process itself involves a loss of much of what we consider attractive. Your body is an exterior and protective casing for your inner functions. If you enjoy decorating it, as you might enjoy decorating your apartment, that's great. But if you find yourself going too far beyond that, you might want to try to challenge the passion.

Extreme Attachment to the Material World. This passion is manifested in several ways.

1. Excessive attachment to relationships. While interacting with and loving others is very important, some people cling to others not out of real love or friendship, but out of a fear of being alone. This type of attachment creates a draining dependency.

2. Attachment to an identity. People define themselves in terms of their professions, avocations, or personalities: "I'm a doctor (a lawyer, a wife and mother, a generous friend)." When the ability to act in the chosen area ends, as is likely when you are facing a dying process, attachment to the role can cause great sorrow.

3. Attachment to the physical body. This attachment can cause difficulty when you're approaching dying. Since we all must leave our bodies behind, people who are at ease with the concept of their soul's continuing seem to leave more comfortably than do those who remain intensely attached to their physical bodies.

Lust. While sex is an important aspect of the expression of some forms of love, lust—sex divorced from relationship—can be confused with love and can be destructive. Sex with a lifelong partner or a new lover can be a beautiful, intimate experience as you approach the end of your life. But trying to deny your upcoming death by engaging in disconnected, casual sex only distracts you from the work of dying, and pushes away the real intimacy you need at this time.

☀ STEP D ☀
Creating Positive Days

The most important needs now are yours. It's up to you to know what you need physically, emotionally, and spiritually and to ask that each of these needs be fulfilled. The things you want now will range from the apparently mundane—such as eating a favorite meal, wearing a special garment, or watching a certain television program—to the most important areas of your life, such as having certain people near you on a daily basis or reading religious or spiritual books. All these needs are important, and all should be met to the extent possible.

Having your needs met will help you create positive days for yourself, days in which you constantly remind yourself of the power of positive thoughts. You can introduce a sense of well-being by telling yourself, as I tell all the patients I counsel, that everything will work out fine. Though that may sound absurd, it's true: all your worries and suffering will pass away in time. Simply close your eyes and say to yourself, "Everything will be okay. At some point, everyone dies. When it's time, it's time." As Hamlet said, "The readiness is all."

You'll face many hardships in the time ahead—you're probably facing them already—but you can keep control of your life and greatly enhance it by focusing on the positive elements in all the areas of your life.

Other people will be an important part of this process. You may want to make peace with certain people, and might need help in creating the circumstances that will make that happen. You will have to talk about things that perhaps you've never been willing to discuss before. Above all, on your positive days especially, enjoy the people in your life. Share reminiscences of times spent together; laugh at old, shared jokes that have grown richer over time. Watch a movie or TV show together. Cherish the time you have together and the bonds that have made these people so important in your life.

Find time to think about doing things you've always wanted to do but never got around to. One of my patients had always dreamed of going to Alaska. He and his wife had talked about it for years, always putting it off. After he was diagnosed with metastatic lung cancer, his family quickly mobilized and put the trip together. Not only was the trip itself a wonderful experience, but planning it and then talking about it afterwards provided him with many hours of pleasure.

Every morning, decide what you want to do that day and which people you want to see or telephone. Make plans for future pleasant days. Perhaps you'll want to visit someone: many people diagnosed with an end-stage disease can still travel. After careful consultation with your physician, you can determine the limits you should put on your activities.

One of my patients found a wonderful way to spend quality time, enjoying himself in good company. Mr. Sachs was an elderly, single man who had spent most of his waking time for many years at a local pub in his small town. He was confined to his hospital bed and a wheelchair in the last two months of his life. I had been concerned about him, knowing he had no family. But every Tuesday and Thursday afternoon his drinking buddy Tom visited with him. They played checkers, watched TV, and talked together for hours at a time. The day Mr. Sachs died, Tom was by his side.

The importance of company can hardly be exaggerated. Whether it's your husband, your mother, or your drinking buddy, spend time with people. Someone once told me that when geese are flying long distances and one of the flock falls to the ground because it's dying, another goose leaves the formation and stays with the dying bird until it exhales it last breath. Only then does the healthy bird rejoin the flock. We would do well to imitate the behavior of these birds.

Each day should offer comfort and care to your body, mind, and spirit. To the extent that you can, you should do something physically pleasurable, even if it is just to sit in the sunlight, watch the rain fall, or eat a favorite food. Give yourself emotional and psychological nourishment, such as talking with loved ones, listening to music, or writing a letter. Address your spiritual needs in whatever way feels good to you.

And have *fun*. Rent old Monty Python films or read P. G. Wodehouse novels. Play Trivial Pursuit with your friends.

Wear outrageous outfits you were afraid to wear before. One of my fondest memories in my work with dying patients is Mrs. McIsaac's hats. Mrs. McIsaac, a fifty-year-old woman, was dying of metastatic breast cancer. She had always been rather conservative, but when she was dying she developed a fondness for wild hats. She had a collection of twenty, and we learned to gauge her mood by which hat she wore. When she was happy, she wore demure, conservative hats. When she was sad or frightened, she wore loud, outrageous hats to cheer herself up. As she approached her final days, very frail and weak, she wore only blue hats. "Blue," she told me, smiling, "is the proper color to wear to heaven." She made of her death and dying a happy and profound game, dressing for the roles she played each day.

CHAPTER 5

Coming to Terms

⇢ STEP E ⇠
Talking to Your Doctor—
The Early Stages

O BTAINING MEDICAL information about your treatment
options, their effects, and their side effects will probably require several meetings with your doctor. When you first get an
end-of-life diagnosis, you begin focusing on gathering information.

When you talk to your doctor during this information-
gathering stage, try to stay focused on getting the medical facts as
clearly as possible. Most doctors are overworked, and many lack
the skills to offer counseling about the emotional aspects of dealing with your illness. As we discuss later in this chapter, you can
get that counseling elsewhere. What you want to know at this
point is the details of your illness.

Gathering information about your condition can help settle
your mind. Understanding specific aspects of your disease and
its prognosis can help you plan for both your immediate and
your distant future. Ask the doctor what, specifically, your diagnosis is, and if you don't understand, ask for very precise clarifi-
cation.

Other Questions

There are a few other questions you may want to ask.

- What are my treatment options?

- What is my prognosis? How long do you think I have to live? While there is no surefire way for your doctor to predict how long you'll live, you can get a general idea of the life span of most people at your stage of disease. You may learn that you have several years to live an active life, and you can make these years great ones.

- Will my prognosis be significantly different if I don't treat the disease medically?

- What are the side effects of the treatments you are suggesting?

- How much time do I have to make up my mind about which treatments to use? If I wait a few weeks to think about it, will I cause the effectiveness of the treatment to diminish?

- Where can I find support groups of people with similar diseases?

- What treatments exist outside those offered by traditional Western medicine and where can I research such alternatives? Since doctors often don't know much about alternative treatments, you may have to search a little further to find answers to this last question. There are excellent books on all the forms of such treatments, most of which include information on how to find practitioners. Check your local bookstore or health food store.

You may also need to search further for answers to some of your questions. Surfing the Internet can be helpful, as can checking out libraries and talking to friends. It may be useful to get a second and even a third medical opinion. Self-help and other support groups, which offer emotional help, can also provide factual help, since their members have faced similar situations to yours. Take as much time as you feel is necessary to help you decide on a treatment plan that is right for you.

Combining Approaches

Many people choose aggressive medical treatments; others choose alternatives, such as herbal medicine or acupuncture; many try a combination of approaches. Often, for example, acupuncture can help relieve the side effects of chemotherapy, as well as address the symptoms of the disease itself. People whose disease is already advanced when it's diagnosed may choose aggressive treatment, or they may decide that this course is unhelpful to them and rely on comfort care only. All these choices are valid. As we saw in Chapter 3, different people with the same diagnosis often make very different decisions about treatments.

In my experience, most patients start off with curative treatments when they are first diagnosed. Surgery, radiation, and systemic treatments such as chemotherapy and tamoxifen therapy all make sense, and your doctor, family, and friends must respect your decision to use them. Depending on the nature of your disease and its prognosis, you may spend several years using these treatments, going into remission for a time, and then using them again.

After a time—and this time will be very different for different people—you may want to take stock of your condition and make new decisions. Your condition will be better or worse, and you will face a new set of choices. (I discuss these choices in Chapter 8.)

In order for you to make the best decisions possible, it's

important to create from the start a good working relationship with your doctor. Often patients expect too much from their doctors, and this, combined with the natural emotions that an end-of-life diagnosis evokes, can cause them to lash out at their doctors. Keep in mind that it's in your interest to avoid creating an adversarial relationship with your health care providers. There are many just demands you can make on them, but you must be able to recognize what those are. I discuss these sorts of demands and how you can best get them met later in this book.

✦ STEP F ✦
Talking to Your Family

Once you know that you have an illness from which you will die, whether in a few months or a few years, it's important to make sure that you spend time with your family and loved ones, both in the near future and in the months or years that remain. For the most part, this time will be unstructured, chosen by everyone involved based on how much you want to see each other, what everyone's time commitments are, and other, individual factors. But you can greatly benefit from having a few structured meetings with particular agendas. I include loved ones because your close friends and your lovers can be as important in your life as your literal family, and sometimes more so.

The initial such meeting should be confined to discussing your treatment options, including their possible and probable outcomes, and to establishing a plan for your remaining time. If you decide you want to create a living will, this is the time to involve your family members. They need to know that you have made a living will and that you want it honored. If you haven't made it yet, your family can see to the details—finding a lawyer, getting the proper forms, and so on. You'll also want to choose a medical proxy—a person who will speak for you and make vital decisions when you are unable to do so on your own—at this time. (I discuss both these issues in Chapter 6, Step I.) Family members should make a plan that includes how financial and legal obligations will be met and who can help support all of you through the process you have entered.

Other questions you want to address include:

- Who will be my primary caregiver?
- What will be the roles and responsibilities of the other loved ones present?
- What additional help can my family request from clergy members, friends, and professional or volunteer caregivers?
- Who will be in charge of searching out options for my care?

Plan to meet regularly to provide support for one another. Acknowledge that you may have many things to say to one another and prepare yourselves to talk personally and openly, in a peaceful and accepting way, about whatever conflicts may remain among you. It is helpful to organize specific times for family meetings in order to facilitate communication.

It's important for you and your family to discuss openly the fact that you will soon be dying. You can all benefit from facing this fact. Inevitably, some of your loved ones will have a harder time dealing with the reality than will others, and they may need some time to accept it.

These situations can be difficult. Often the dying person is reluctant to upset loved ones by speaking openly of death; sometimes the loved ones are hesitant to speak. But the subject must be broached by somebody. I've noticed that people often approach their dying as they approached their living. Those who have been good at communicating throughout life usually continue to share their feelings with those close to them. Less communicative people tend to be less comfortable with the process of sharing their thoughts about an end-of-life situation. Still, behavior is not etched in stone. I've seen many previously uncommunicative people open up astoundingly to their loved ones at this time, achieving an eloquence and clarity they have never before had.

In future family meetings, you'll want to get past the practical concerns and discuss aspects of your relationship that have been difficult. Many important issues can finally be resolved at this time.

Sometimes you'll want to talk with people about your difficulties—the pain you're in, your frustrations at decreasing mobility, your fears of dying. Your loved ones will have to adapt to your new situation. You'll need a lot of rest; they'll have to get used to sitting quietly with you for long periods of time. They'll need to learn to accept your withdrawals without feeling hurt or impatient. Sometimes you'll find the people you love trying. Some people simply can't contain their expressions of grief. While you'll all need a lot of honest sharing of emotions, you may not have the energy to constantly deal with other people's emotional outbursts. When someone is overly emotional, you or one of the others around you should explain that this reaction is draining on everyone and, if the outbursts continue, they need to be asked to leave the room.

Some families will not be interested in using a formal approach, but they can use some of the techniques on their own in a less formal way.

You may need to help your family along, since even those who are better able to face the situation may find it difficult to talk with you about it. You can help them by broaching the subject yourself, saying something like, "This is a scary and difficult time for all of us. Let me tell you how scared I am about what's happening to me, and please tell me what *you're* feeling, too." Address some of the fears they may have: "This is changing our lives, isn't it? Does it make you as anxious as it makes me?" Talk about your treatment options and ask for their advice: be sure to consider the impact the treatment can have on all your lives—the weakness caused by radiation, for example, or the nausea from chemotherapy.

Your family members will probably respond in different ways, based on their own styles. Some people are very private, preferring to keep emotions to themselves. Others see showing emotion as a sign of weakness. It's important that you allow everyone—including yourself—whatever time is needed to become comfortable with your situation. On the other hand, don't let "giving ourselves time to deal with it" become an excuse for *never* dealing with it. Sooner or later, you're all going to have to face the fear, sadness, grief, anger, and feelings of hopelessness that confront dying people and those who love them. The more you, or any of your loved ones, can facilitate honest communication, the easier this difficult situation will become.

Family Meetings

There are some formal techniques that members of your family can use to help them deal with you and your circumstances. One of the best of these, developed by Dr. N. Michael Murphy, a pioneer in the U.S. hospice movement, is a five-part technique that guides families in their communication with a loved one who is dying.

According to Dr. Murphy, a family meeting of some sort is especially important for families that have had difficulty communicating. It is helpful to have someone facilitate the meeting, which should involve all family members, including children and grandchildren. (Dr. Murphy's model addresses only the traditional family, but can be applied equally to chosen families—friends and lovers who are often as important and sometimes even more important to a person than are the people legally defined as family.) The first part of the family meeting can begin with what Dr. Murphy calls "the story of the wound": the dying person tells the story of the illness from beginning to end. This uninterrupted narrative gives the family a sense of how the dying person is experiencing this powerful time of life. In some cases, this is the first time a family member gets to speak without others' placing their opinions and needs into the discussion.

The facilitator then directs the conversation toward worries and fears, allowing the dying person to talk about concerns and love for individual family members. These are often deep-rooted feelings, and expressing them can lead to healing and closure on important issues. In Dr. Murphy's words, "Surprisingly enough, the disappointments, disillusionments and resentments when voiced can be let go and room is made for the expression of vulnerability, tenderness and love."*

The third area of family discussion, called "roots," allows the dying person to talk about the past, including other deaths. Dr. Murphy points out that "reflections about parents, siblings and growing up often reveal continuing pain from deaths unmourned and loving words unspoken." Facing the issue of previous deaths within the family can help allow the person to die in peace, having addressed hidden worries and fears. It helps create a context of continuity: one sees one's own dying in relation to other deceased family members.

In the next stage of the family meeting, "the family speaks," everyone talks about the dying person, sharing both good times

---

* This and the following quotations are from Dr. Murphy's *When All Is Said and Done* Study Guide (Watertown, Mass.: Vox Populi Productions, 1995).

and hard times, with emphasis on how advancing illness is affecting the family members and their own hopes and fears. Family secrets, such as alcoholism, abuse, and shame, may come up in the context of a lifelong relationship's coming to an end.

The meeting closes with a positive statement, in which family members can, Dr. Murphy explains, "in their own way bless the dying person." The blessing need not have any specific ritualistic connotation; rather, it creates a moment to embrace the dying person with a good wish.

This open, honest conversation can have a powerful effect on everyone involved, as described by Dr. Murphy: "The stories that we are told are important, but it goes far beyond words said. It is as if the intention and willingness to be present, open and truthful about what lies within the soul somehow makes this process work, whether words are spoken or not."

Your Treatment Choice

A vital function of communicating with family members involves allowing you to choose your own course of medical treatment and be certain that it is carried out. When you have all finished discussing choices of treatment, the decisions belong solely to you. It is important that everyone else respect these decisions and implement them. If you request comfort care versus medical treatment directed toward curing disease, some people will be horrified and confused. Even if they appear to respect your desires, they may well speak differently away from you: "We can't just let her die!" "We have to do something for him." These are very common sentiments. Your loved ones need to understand that at the appropriate time, a treatment plan based solely on comfort care *is* doing something for you. Helping you die peacefully, once you've made that choice, is one of the most loving acts possible. Family members need to let you know that they respect all your requests, even if they are struggling with these choices.

When your medical condition worsens, your family members and your designated health care proxy (who will be in charge of communicating with the doctors and health care workers) must be your advocates, interpreting your advance directives. If you want comfort care only, then your proxy must make certain that you get only care-based treatment. Your family will need courage and strength to fight anything that is contrary to your wishes.

Connecting with Children

Discussing family dynamics at the time of dying would be incomplete without addressing the issue of children's involvement in the dying process. Our culture has historically attempted to shield children from dying. In many other cultures, dying is understood as a natural process, and children aren't kept away from the bedsides of dying relatives.

If you want children to be around you, they should be allowed to visit if they wish. Having children around, especially children you love, is a tender reminder of life's continuity and can be a wonderful part of your dying experience.

It is helpful for parents to prepare children for the fact that a person they love dearly will be very sick and weak for a time and won't be around for as long as the child might wish. Children need help coming to terms with the death of a loved one. Honest, direct communication, geared toward their level of understanding, can help children deal with the difficult reality ahead. In the long run, being involved with you during your end-of-life illness will probably be a very positive experience for the children you love. They'll have much less trouble dealing with death in the rest of their lives if dying is not hidden from them now.

What *isn't* good for children is seeing adult fears about dying and having people mysteriously disappear from their lives without being able to say good-bye. I know many adults who as children experienced the death of a close friend or family member. Those who were involved in the process—visiting the dying person, helping in caretaking, and so on—are far more comfortable with the idea of their own and others' dying than are those who were kept away from the knowledge that the person was dying or from interactions at the later stages of dying. Although adults in the former group still grieve and still have fears and questions, they can work with their feelings. The others tend to have deeper fears and far more of a tendency to remain in denial about dying and death.

☀ STEP G ☀
Coming to Terms with This Reality

The first thing you'll need to realize when you have an advanced illness is that you need time to adapt to your new circumstances. On some level you're trying to accept the unacceptable. Your mind is rebelling against the facts being presented to you. Your fear of dying causes you to grasp at life. Yet some deeper part of you is struggling to accept what is occurring now. If you let it, that part can eventually overcome all your resistances and help you embrace the experience.

Take it slowly. Don't try to deal with situations or events that haven't yet arisen and may never arise. The danger at this particular moment is of being overwhelmed, especially by possibilities. It's hard not to obsess—to visualize with terror the process of dying, the pain and helplessness of the end as you might perceive it now. Many people are deeply unhappy at this point and feel particularly isolated living with an end-of-life state.

Sadly, such feelings are often reflections of real experience. Many people with advanced illness are abandoned by friends and family members. One cause of this reaction is a fear of contagion. With diseases such as AIDS, people tend to exaggerate the danger of contagion, and even with noncontagious illnesses, such as cancers, ignorance can cause terror. But the primary fear goes deeper than that. Many people treat dying itself as a contagious disease. Steeped in denial of death, people often flee the reminder of their own mortality that they see in a dying loved one.

Doctors also often disappear from a dying person's life. The primary care doctors who have worked with the patient may leave the picture once they've referred the patient to specialists who deal with the particular disease.

It may be helpful to keep this in mind from the beginning of your diagnosis. Try to talk with the people close to you right away, to prevent as much as possible being isolated as you get closer to dying. If your loved ones are prepared for the situation, they're less likely to hide from it when the time comes. As with any situation requiring dramatic change—moving, for example, or going on a long trip—the more planning you can do, the better prepared everyone will be.

So, make the plans you need to make and help your loved ones make their plans. Remember the sage advice of Alcoholics Anonymous: change what can be changed, accept what can't be changed, and be wise enough to see which is which. And having done the planning you can, don't obsess. Move yourself and your loved ones back into the present, the only clear reality. All you can know with any certainty in such difficult times is *right now*, this very moment. Practice coming back to the present. Choose to make the most of this moment. Be with people you care about. If you wish, spend short periods of time alone in an environment you find particularly peaceful and supportive. Do not become isolated, however. Too much time alone can be destructive now.

If you're someone who lives alone and doesn't have many friends to turn to for support, this might be a good time to seek people out. There are support groups for people with many life-threatening illnesses, and these can be tremendously helpful. People who are going through what you're going through can be a great help to you, and you can be a great help to them. You might have casual friends and acquaintances who would be glad to offer support if they knew you wanted it. The Internet offers chat lines and forums for people in various life situations, including illnesses. If you are religious, you might turn to your local church or synagogue.

You can do other things to keep from obsessing about the future. Read, watch television shows you particularly enjoy, or work on your hobbies. If you don't have any hobbies, now might be a good time to start one. You can participate in many things, from stamp collecting to listening to music, even when you're confined to your bed.

Once you've absorbed the impact of your diagnosis, you can begin to think through the future. But be sure to do so in a disciplined, orderly way. Don't take on everything at once: sit down with a pen and paper or your computer and develop a preliminary plan that describes how you want to spend your remaining time. Who are the people you want to spend time with now? What would you like to do now? Where do you want to spend your remaining time? Do you want to update your will? How do you plan to resolve your financial obligations? What emotional, psychological, and spiritual issues would you like to resolve before you die? All of these questions require time to answer: don't rush yourself through them.

One thing that can help is keeping a journal in which you

explore your feelings and thoughts and acknowledge and fulfill any desires that emerge. Pay close attention to specific issues that are unsettling and need your attention. Slowly, a solid plan for what you want to do with the months or years you have left can take form. You will benefit from getting help with, or talking with others about, resolving difficult issues.

Major Issues

Most people need to resolve issues in four major areas.

1. They need to deal with questions surrounding family and relationships.

2. They need to determine what to do about their jobs.

3. They need to grapple with the specifics of declining health.

4. They need to look at spiritual questions—the meaning of this life and if, or how, their consciousness lives on.

List any major obstacles that exist for you in any of these areas. Do any of your past relationships remain unresolved? Do you still have financial problems to address? Are you still fighting with yourself over decisions you have made about your health? Are you worried about the well-being of your loved ones? It is time to resolve as best you can all that you ran from in the past.

Few of the questions you come up with will be new: chances are you have been dealing with the same issues throughout your life. What changes now is the balance. If you look carefully and balance your logical worries with a sense of calm, you'll see that there is a shift in what is important in you. This shift will help you reassess your old priorities and see life in a new way. Some of the things that once seemed crucial will diminish in importance;

some things that you kept on the back burner will now take on major significance.

To plan realistically it is important, practically and ethically, for your doctor to reveal all the medical facts to you. I have seen people who were devastated when they heard their diagnosis, but who fully recovered their clarity and equilibrium within weeks and were very much in control of their lives once again. If your doctor seems evasive, press for further information and be clear that you are ready to handle whatever you're told.

Believe it or not, you still have many good, even wonderful days to live. Soon you'll discover that you've accepted what you're going through. You may find that you even look forward with a peaceful feeling to what lies ahead.

⟡ STEP H ⟡
Seeking Counseling and Support

In earlier parts of this century, and indeed throughout medical tradition, the physician was both healer and, to some degree, counselor. This is rarely the case today, since doctors are not usually trained to provide such counseling. Most people who are facing dying will have to take the initiative to get counseling or have their loved ones find counseling for them.

You will probably need to approach your doctors and their support staff with specific questions.

- Where can I find someone skilled in short-term counseling, particularly someone who has worked with people facing death?

- Where have other people with my medical diagnosis found helpful counseling?

- Are there any self-help groups in the area that can help me?

If your doctor can't answer these questions, there are other avenues you can take. In most communities you can find counselors who are experienced in working with people who have advanced illnesses. Local hospitals, clergy, and mental health groups (which should be listed in your Yellow Pages) can give you the names of such therapists.

Once you've gotten the names of some counselors, you'll want to interview them. People are often hesitant to do this, but the wrong counselor will only worsen your fears. Above all, you need a counselor who is comfortable with death and dying. If the person seems to be pitying you, it's a bad sign. Compassion is fine; pity is a dodge. You want someone able to focus matter-of-factly on your current situation and your fears and concerns.

You may need just a few sessions to help clarify specific issues, or you may find you need a longer time and more support with the whole process. As helpful as a counselor can be, remember that in our current medical system the doctors, not the counselors, make treatment decisions. Therefore, you'll want to make sure that all your personal health care decisions are communicated clearly to your doctor (see Chapter 8, Step O).

Fortunately, the medical establishment is beginning to recognize that medical students need to be trained in counseling and communication skills. I hope that widespread training in caring for the dying will become part of all medical training in the near future.

CHAPTER 6

Practical Matters

❖ STEP I ❖
Selecting Advance Directives

ONE OF the most important things you can do to keep control of your end-of-life situation and make your own dying
peaceful is to create documents that spell out what life-prolonging measures you do and don't want taken. In addition, you'll
want to identify someone—a proxy—who will speak on your
behalf in the event that you're not able to make your wishes
known. Communicating your desires to your doctor and your
family is also critical to make certain that the wishes you spell
out in your documents are followed.

Without written documentation, you are helpless against
doctors or family members who don't respect your wishes. I remember too vividly the last days of my grandmother Bobby. I
knew Bobby well when I was a child. She was vibrant and full of
life. She told me that when her time came, she wanted to go out
with no fuss, with no machines keeping her body alive artificially. To her, this was so logical that she assumed everyone else
would agree: she trusted that common sense would prevail when
she reached her dying.

When she was seventy-eight, she began to exhibit the signs of
dementia, and within a few years the disease had taken over. She
was placed in a nursing home in 1975. She lived there for years in
a state of deep confusion, unable to recognize her children and

grandchildren. Her condition remained essentially unchanged until one morning when she began to develop labored breathing. Sensing a change in her medical condition, the staff quickly placed her in an ambulance to go to the nearest city hospital emergency room. There, a medical resident recognized her breathing difficulty and immediately placed a tube in her mouth, through her throat, and into her lungs. The tube attached her to an artificial breathing machine called a ventilator. She was then tethered to the machine, with her arms and legs tied to restrain her. This is a common procedure, as patients will attempt to remove breathing tubes, intravenous tubes, and other apparatus in their confusion and pain.

My brother called me, upset with the decision to place this ninety-four-year-old woman on a ventilator. I was shocked. After everything I had seen in my medical career, I could not bear the thought of my grandmother being attached to this machine, restrained and suffering, when I knew it could do her no good. I immediately called my mother and uncle. They didn't feel competent to challenge the medical authorities. "We're letting the doctors do what they think is best," they told me.

I then called Bobby's supervising medical doctor, who explained that when she came to the emergency room there were no advance directives with her, so they were legally obligated to do everything to keep her alive. To get her off the ventilator, Bobby's children would have to file a complicated appeal, which they wouldn't do. My uncle did, however, request the hospital not to resuscitate his mother in the future, if she were ever to get off the breathing machine. A hospital nurse documented his request over the phone, although everyone was convinced that Bobby would shortly die. Surprisingly, within several weeks, her breathing difficulty cleared, and she was weaned off the breathing machine and sent back to her nursing home.

Several days later, Bobby's breathing once again slowed

down, and the nursing home staff rushed her off to a different hospital's emergency room. My uncle's request had not been placed in Bobby's permanent nursing home chart, so she was once again attached to a breathing machine and tied down.

Bobby had a strong heart, which kept her alive, alone in a strange hospital room, attached to a bunch of machines, for over six and a half months. Finally, mercifully, she died.

When Bobby was well, little was known about written wills and advance directives. Had she fallen ill a few years later, she probably would have documented her wishes. Fortunately, such documents are far more common today.

Advance directives are written instructions placed in two main documents, a living will and a health care proxy. A living will contains future requests regarding medical treatment, and a health care proxy assigns someone to make future decisions in case the person becomes unable to do so. I will outline the standard living will, a living will with a do-not-resuscitate order, and a living will that incorporates refusal of other specific treatments.

Creating a living will and health care proxy when you are well is a first step in trying to communicate your choices in medical care. Such documents can help prevent misunderstanding and unwanted medical intervention. Good and frequent communication with your primary physician, who will be managing your medical condition, is crucial here. Your doctor must know you well enough to know how serious you are about your wishes, and you must be very clear with your doctor about which procedures you do and don't want done at different stages of your illness.

Living Will—Standard Form

Living wills, which vary from state to state, address some of the treatments you may want to decline at a specific time in life. By reviewing the sample documents in Appendix 3, you can get an idea of the specific treatments listed in a living will as well as the specific terms for implementation of the will. Like most living wills, these samples state that resuscitation or life-prolonging measures may be declined when a person has "an incurable or irreversible mental or physical condition with no reasonable expectation of recovery."

LIVING WILL — DO NOT RESUSCITATE

The language in the sample standard forms is fine as far as it goes. The problem is that it doesn't go far enough. The decision as to when someone has "an incurable and irreversible condition" is currently left to the doctor in charge. That doctor may argue that treatments always offer the possibility, however slim, of curing the disease and reversing dying. So if you're certain at any point that you don't want to prolong your life artificially, you need something stronger than the standard living will. You'll want to upgrade your living will by adding to it a clear statement, known as a DNR (do not resuscitate), that you do not want to be resuscitated under any circumstances. This request removes the need for the doctor or anyone else to interpret vague phrasing. It states that you do not want your failing heart restarted with CPR or failed breathing restored with a mechanical breathing machine. This crucial change clearly says that no one is to decide on any treatment other than what you have requested. The doctor does not have to judge what constitutes a curable or irreversible state. For example, the DNR in Appendix 3 reads "Do not resuscitate the person named above." The DNR request could not be any clearer; once the primary physician enters a DNR order in the chart, there is a good chance that it will be respected, even in crisis. It takes planning to prepare such a document and have it entered into your hospital chart. The decision to change your living will to include a DNR requires a great deal of thought. Do-not-resuscitate orders vary from state to state, and they must always be signed by a physician. There is a separate DNR form used for nonhospital situations (for example, if you are dying at home), but each hospital also has its own DNR form. Many of the specifics will be covered in Step M, "Balancing Cure and Care."

Sadly, a DNR isn't foolproof either. Doctors don't always enter these requests into their charts. A 1995 study published in the *Journal of the American Medical Association* found that nearly half the wishes of all dying patients who asked their doctors to issue do-not-resuscitate orders were ignored.* This study shocked many people, who began to question the value of filling out advance directives at all. However, the combination of an advance directive and good communication with your doctor and family makes it far more likely that your wishes will be honored. Even a directive by itself significantly increases your chances of getting the care you want, which is far better than no chance at all.

LIVING WILL — OTHER SPECIFIC TREATMENTS

Other treatments that need to be clarified in a written advance directive, leaving no room for interpretation, are artificial nutrition, artificial hydration, and antibiotic usage. Artificial nutrition means feeding the body through tubes when it can no longer take nutrition orally on its own: the most common method is to place tubes through the nose, down the throat, and into the stomach.

Providing artificial nutrition makes sense when it is directed toward recovery and when there is hope that the person can eventually have the tube removed and eat normally. However,

---

* The Support Principal Investigators, "A Controlled Trial to Improve Care for Seriously Ill Hospital Patients," *Journal of the American Medical Association* 277, no. 20 (November 22, 1995).

feeding tubes are extremely uncomfortable and make little sense for someone who is ready to accept dying.

A more permanent form of feeding tube is the gastric tube. Unlike the other tubes, which involve no surgery, it's inserted surgically through the abdomen into the stomach. It cannot be removed without another operation. On the surface, this may seem appealing. It isn't nearly as uncomfortable as the tube that's placed down the throat and into the stomach. The person can walk around with a fair degree of comfort. There's the danger of infection that exists in all surgeries, and some discomfort from the operation, but aside from that it isn't very physically painful. So you may want your advance directive to state that you want a gastric tube if you stop being able to eat.

However, it's not always that simple. I've known numerous patients who've had gastric tubes inserted and regretted it later, even though it added several months to their lives. One problem is the quality of life in those months. If you're close enough to death that you stop wanting food, it means that the disease process is ready to play itself out, with all the pain and discomfort that terminal illness usually brings. You may find yourself trading a relatively painless death for a much more uncomfortable one.

But I think the problems with gastric tubes go deeper than that. People tend to choose feeding tubes or other interventions because they want to believe they can defeat death. But deep down they know they can't really do that. They tend to feel that they're in a dreary limbo, not dead but no longer really belonging to life. "Good Time Charlie," one of the patients I worked with at the VA hospital, brought this home to me very clearly. He had never been counseled about the tube—they told him it was a good idea, he said fine, and he had the surgery. He would walk around, smoking his cigarettes. He made a big ritual of his feeding: whenever he had to feed himself, he paid great attention to preparing the tube. But it wasn't a joyful ritual. He seemed to be constantly brooding. He talked to me several times about the tube. "It just doesn't feel right," he would say. "I'm alive, but I'm not supposed to be alive. I don't feel like I'm living, just like I'm passing time with this thing in me. I wish I hadn't done it." Finally, one day, he just clamped the tube shut and stopped using it. "That's it," he told me. A few days later, he died.

During all my talks with Charlie, I felt strongly that he had been shortchanged. No one had discussed the tube with him in advance. No one had helped him explore how he might feel about prolonging his life in this highly artificial way. Perhaps if someone had done so, he still would have chosen to have the procedure, but at least then he would have been prepared for the terrible hollowness he felt during those last weeks of his life. Or perhaps he would have realized that his own sense of what was natural would be violated by the tube, as ultimately it was.

Of course, Charlie did end up making his own decision; he closed off the tube. But for most people, such an action would be much harder than choosing not to have a feeding tube inserted in the first place. Because it's so much more active, closing the tube seems closer to suicide.

Another intervention is artificial hydration—placing fluids in the body, usually sterile water and sugar solutions through an IV (a small tube inserted into a vein in the arm or neck). Intravenous fluid is routinely used when the body cannot take in enough fluid by mouth. Again, it makes sense when there is hope of recovery. When you're preparing to die, however, intravenous fluids are unnecessary and cause discomfort and agitation. Ice chips, as well as wet washcloths applied to the lips, will help with some of the discomfort of dehydration, but when it is time to die the body does not need much hydration.

This is a crucial point. Loved ones usually misunderstand and think the dying person is suffering terrible pangs of hunger and thirst. People do not starve to death when they stop eating food or die of thirst when they stop drinking water. The body slows down in a very fixed and natural way at the end of life. In most cases, people stop eating and drinking precisely because they feel no more need to do so. They do not suffer pangs of hunger or thirst.

Often, dying people are given antibiotics, medications that fight infection-causing germs (bacteria). They're an excellent tool for people who will recover from their illnesses. But when you're preparing to die in a comfortable setting, antibiotics may not be necessary except to control a painful local infection. Often people who are dying get pneumonia, and nowadays doctors tend to give them antibiotics. In the past, though, pneumonia was known as "the old people's friend," because it brought death in a relatively comfortable way. So again, if you get antibiotics for pneumonia at a very advanced stage in your illness, you might be setting yourself up for a lingering and uncomfortable death later.

CHOICES

You should ask yourself five routine questions when facing an end-of-life situation.

At this point in my life, taking into account my total condition if my bodily functions were to continue slowing down, do I want:

❑ Yes ❑ No **1.** To be attached to a mechanical breathing machine?

❑ Yes ❑ No **2.** To have my heart resuscitated with medications and mechanical methods?

❑ Yes ❑ No **3.** To be fed with a feeding tube?

❑ Yes ❑ No **4.** To be given fluid hydration with intravenous lines?

❑ Yes ❑ No **5.** To be given antibiotics?

If you are ready to die and don't want your life prolonged by mechanical breathing machines, nutritional and hydration tubes, drugs and mechanical techniques to reverse heart failure, or antibiotics, you should change your standard living will to a request that does not require interpretation.

You can do this with advance directives in any of the five standard areas. You need to analyze each of these areas, if possible before you're in a hospital setting. Although family members and doctors will all have their own opinions, which are worth listening to, you must ultimately trust your own internal wisdom in making these decisions.

Expressing your wishes doesn't mean you have to decide *not* to have certain treatments. In some cases, patients and their families have to be adamant about their desire to continue medical care. In *Dying at Home,* Andrea Sankar tells of one woman whose husband had clearly stated his wishes to be resuscitated if it would save his life. The doctor insisted on withdrawing all treatment, despite the wife's objections. Because she was there and able to fight for what she knew her husband wanted, the doctor gave in and performed the procedure.*

That last sentence is crucial. The woman fought for the procedure *because her husband had clearly let her know, in advance, that this was what he wanted.* This is far different from the more common situation in which family members defy the patient's wish to be free from such interventions. Whatever scenario you choose, you have to let your loved ones know your wishes well in advance, and you have to let them know that you expect them to honor and, if need be, fight for those wishes.

Many variables are involved in thinking through the dying process, but ultimately what you need to decide is whether you

---

* Andrea Sankar, *Dying at Home: A Family Guide for Caregiving* (New York: Bantam Books, 1995), pp. 23–24.

want further medical treatment directed toward cure, or simply comfort-care therapy, at a given time. Both decisions are equally valid and must be respected.

Remember that an advance directive is never irreversible. For example, if you feel on a given day that you would want to be resuscitated and artificially fed because deep in your heart you still hope there's a chance of recovery or for any other reason, you can change your living will, notifying your family and your health care proxy both in writing and orally. Usually, however, by the time you've done all the preparation and contemplation to become ready for dying, you won't change your decision to focus only on care-based treatment.

Your Health Care Proxy

Another important issue is who will be your health care proxy in the event that you can no longer speak for yourself. You need to choose this person very carefully. It should be someone who understands your philosophy of living and dying and who will be able to accurately translate your wishes about the specifics of your treatment when you're unable to express them yourself. Make certain you choose someone who is willing to take on such a responsibility and who has a forceful enough personality to fight for your wishes. This may be the person who is closest to you, but it may not. Your husband may be very loving and supportive, but not a great fighter. Your wife may agree with your choice intellectually, but have emotional difficulty with it. It may be too difficult for a parent to make a decision not to prolong a beloved child's life.

If the person you choose for your proxy isn't related to you by blood or marriage, you need to be doubly careful to create as legally binding a proxy as possible. Gay and lesbian couples, as well as unmarried heterosexual couples, are especially vulnerable in this area. Such partners have no legal status, and family members are often hostile toward unorthodox relationships. Your family members must respect your choice of proxy, as they must respect all the decisions you make surrounding your dying.

A long legal battle that took place in the 1980s and early 1990s illustrates what can happen if you don't have a proxy and your family is hostile toward others in your life. Sharon Kowalski and Karen Thompson were lovers who had lived together for several years when Kowalski was injured in a car accident that left her permanently disabled—she could no longer talk or move. Both she and Thompson wanted to remain together, and Thompson had a house built especially to accommodate Kowalski's disabilities. Kowalski's parents objected because of their disapproval of lesbianism. It took eight years and $220,000 in legal fees before the courts allowed Kowalski to live with Thompson.* Kowalski had been young and healthy before being suddenly disabled by the accident. With a serious disease, you know the possibilities ahead of time and can prevent a similar situation from occurring to you.

✦ STEP J ✦
Considering Other Practical Concerns

You'll want to deal with other details at this time also. It's a good idea at some point to look at everything in your life—all your projects, plans, relationships, even future events in which you won't participate—and clearly state how you want your affairs handled after you're gone. There are usually legal, financial, and business relationships that must be clarified. There may be projects you want a particular person, or people, to finish after you

---

* Linda Wong, "Thompson and Kowalski Still Need Help," *Sojourner*, February 1993, p. 10.

die. You may have special wishes about weddings, birthdays, or other celebrations that you want fulfilled. Based on your decisions about how you want to spend your remaining time, you may choose to concentrate on different aspects of your life. I've seen some people go back to college or continuing-education centers to study subjects they've been interested in for a long time, while others have continued doing the things they've always enjoyed most.

Often people decide at this time to reevaluate and restructure relationships. You might want to reconnect with old friends or work out long-standing problems with someone in your family or workplace. One patient I worked with, Mr. Anton, was a successful businessman who had loved his work and prospered in it. He had enjoyed most of his business relationships, with one glaring exception—a fifteen-year feud with a former partner. He telephoned the man and made peace with him. "The business world has been good to me," he told me. "I want to be at peace with it now."

Some people facing an incurable illness decide to let go of superficial relationships, particularly those based on gossip or pettiness, so they can focus their time on the things that really matter to them. Throughout the process of facing your dying, you may find that your new situation teaches you to arrange your priorities differently.

Writing Your Will

If you haven't yet made out a will, now is the time to do it. It's important to have a will, even if the money will eventually go where you want it anyway—to your spouse or children. Without a will there may be long delays in settling your estate, and the government may end up with a larger part than it would otherwise. (The extent to which this happens varies from state to state.)

Even if you're dying broke, a will can be a good idea. Bequests may be emotionally if not financially significant. You might want a favorite niece to have your childhood copy of *Little Women* or your bowling buddy to have your bowling ball. Some of these things you can distribute now, while you're still alive, but others you might want to put into a will. My coauthor had a dear friend who died of breast cancer while still in her thirties. She did not have much money, and most of what she had went, naturally, to her husband and their two small children. But she did leave a thousand dollars to my coauthor, with the stipulation that she spend it "on something fun." My coauthor used it for a trip to Switzerland, where a close mutual friend lived.

There are other advantages to making a will: it ensures that your loved ones will be looked after to whatever extent your money can bring that about, and it may prevent quarrels among relatives over your goods.

Be careful, however, to use your will for positive ends. Don't try to get even with a relative you've quarreled with. You want to end your life resolving old hostilities, not perpetuating them.

And don't make your will a major obsession. Think about it carefully, talk it over with your lawyer and trusted friends or relatives, write it, and put it aside. You can always make changes, of course, but if you find yourself changing your will every other day, you're diverting energy that you need for more important things. Even writing a will can become a means of grasping!

Other Details

A multitude of details about the dying process itself need to be addressed—where it should take place (see Chapter 9, Step Q);

the people you want present when you die; and your funeral arrangements (see Chapter 10, Step X).

In the face of all that is happening now, it's easy to forget important aspects of life that you will leave unfinished but do not have to abandon. Take a look around you, and at a time when you're feeling calm, make a list of the projects that are important to you. Decide realistically what you can and cannot do. List those you can do in the near future, and make another list of those you probably won't get to. Think about whether there are people you could ask to complete your projects or to look after them for you. Keep in mind that your decisions are your own, to be made in your own way and with your own style.

One of my patients, Mr. Ray, had always been compulsive about all the details of his life. Facing his death, he decided to spend his last six months studying spiritual works. "I want to return to the heart of God," he told me passionately. The practical details that had consumed so much of his life suddenly meant nothing to him.

Another patient, Mrs. Blair, chose to spend her final eighteen months completing community projects, such as building a food bank through her church. She spent very little time with her family or friends, but happily immersed herself in fund-raising and doing other work on the projects that had given her so much joy in her life.

Many people decide to leave expressions of their thoughts so that after they have died, their loved ones have intimate records of them. These take the form of poems, letters, or audio- or videotapes. One of my younger patients, a forty-eight-year-old man dying of stomach cancer, worked with a music therapist and composed a song for his wife. She taped him singing it to her. After his death she played the song for me, and I could feel his presence in the music. It was a wonderful gift to leave.

Other people feel that they don't need to leave records for the adults in their lives, since they are able to say all they wanted to them in person, but want to leave messages for children. Young children might not understand or remember the situation: messages for them can make a difference when they're in their teens and better able to grasp the meaning.

A particularly moving story is that of David Taub, a thirty-eight-year-old man dying of metastatic colon cancer. He had two daughters, aged six and eight. He spent days composing letters to the girls. He wanted his wife to give each girl her letter when she turned fourteen. He thought this was an age at which a child could understand such a letter. He showed me parts of these letters, which were moving expressions of how the girls were in no way responsible for his death and of how he would be thinking of them forever.

The practical concerns of people facing end-of-life situations are as varied as those of anyone else. You can choose the issues most important to you and work on them as you see fit. Tying up your loose ends is a major contribution to letting go of life peacefully.

CHAPTER 7

Your Spiritual Destiny

➺ STEP K ➻
Examining Spiritual Views on Living and Dying

T HROUGHOUT YOUR life, but especially when facing an end-of-life situation, you have the ability to explore and develop a relationship with the possibility of your own particular spiritual destiny. Spirituality, as I define it in this book, is a person's individual understanding of, and relationship to, a higher power—a vital source of energy or force that connects with all of existence. Few people in their daily lives stop and think about life as a spiritual journey. They go through the motions of religion or of disbelief or simply go on with the business of living. Others do look at the larger cosmic questions. They periodically reflect on the overall meaning of life and of their particular lives; they ponder their beliefs about God, religion, and what exists after this life; they ask themselves whether they are living according to their own spiritual and moral convictions.

Rarely have I seen a dying person who hasn't struggled with these questions. At this point, if never before, you'll find yourself asking questions like: What have I done with my life and what can I still do with it? Is there a purpose in my life's struggle?

Some—in my experience, a very few—patients are hard-core atheists, and for them, those questions are enough. The rest go on with other questions. What is the nature of the next phase of my existence? What is my relationship with spirit or divinity?

Do I need spiritual counseling or assistance now? What are my spiritual needs at this time? What happens to me after I die? Where did I come from? What is "soul," and does it continue on in an eternal life? Is there a higher power to which we're all connected?

If these questions emerge for you, grappling with them is an important part of your life, which, now, is your dying process. Explore your spiritual beliefs. Ferret out any beliefs that may have always been part of your being but have lain quietly within you. You may find unexpected resources there, and you may want to share your experiences with those around you.

I realize that there are people uninterested in developing a spiritual perspective on life or on their own dying experiences. If you're among these, this chapter may not interest you, and you should feel free to skip the rest of it and move on to the steps in the program that are more useful to you. But I've found in working with people facing their own dying that this situation is atypical. Most of the patients I've worked with have told me that once they entered the dying process, they realized that life and all its experiences had meaning for them and that investigating this meaning was important to them.

A Higher Power?

Being spiritual doesn't mean believing in a particular religion or even a particular definition of God. One of my friends, a man in his eighties in an early stage of prostate cancer, does a lot of thinking about life and death. He explained his concept of spirituality as a belief in the importance of goodness, which he has attempted to follow in his life as his guiding principle. He doesn't feel any connection to any higher power, nor does he believe that the good or evil people do in this life have any reverberations in a future one: he is convinced that the soul dies with the body. For him, spirituality means doing good work that has helped the community.

If you do have a belief in some higher power, it can be a great source of comfort to you now. I've seen a strong sense of gratitude and acceptance in dying people who have discovered their own belief in an eternal higher power. Sometimes this is an extension of a long-held belief, as it was in the case of one of the patients at the VA, Mr. Ives. I remember him vividly because of the beautiful calm I saw in his face when I first met him. He was seventy years old, bedridden by advanced metastatic bladder cancer. I introduced myself to him and asked if he understood what was going on.

He smiled gently at me. "What's going on is what's going on. I trust in God's plan to take me back to his heart. No problem, Doc." As we talked more over several days, I learned where that deep faith came from. He was a black man who had grown up in the south, where he had experienced ugly racism and violence. But his parents were strong Baptists who believed in a loving God and passed that belief on to their children. This belief had helped him deal with all the tribulations of his life, and it did not desert him now. He talked of "making his way back to heaven" and of accepting "whatever God's plan for all of us was." In the weeks I saw him, his faith never wavered.

A similar belief sustained Mrs. Barbutto, a Roman Catholic woman who was slowing down because of advancing diabetes and heart disease. Her condition had not been defined as terminal, but she understood that she was not likely to have many years left. "I know I'm not actually dying," she told me, "but I think about death a great deal." In the past she had worried about dying, but as she came closer to its reality, this was changing. "Strangely enough, as I grow weaker, I worry less." Then she looked at me for a moment and said, "You worry a lot, don't you?"

I was taken by surprise. "I've struggled all my life with worry and tried hard to change it," I admitted.

"You can change it," she told me. "Remember that, whatever religion you grew up with, there's only one God, and God with his helpers looks after everyone. I just put my focus on God, and my worries become his problem. It makes whatever happens to me next make a lot of sense."

For people like Mr. Ives and Mrs. Barbutto, faith is a given, a resource they use all their lives. Others, however, may need to search for their spiritual identity. Often people who have been away from religion and spirituality realize that the beliefs of their childhood have remained buried deep inside them, and are there to help them now.

Charlie, a frank, opinionated, elderly man dying of prostate cancer, prided himself on always speaking his mind. One day we were talking together in his room when the hospital's priest came in and introduced himself. Charlie glared at him. "The last time I went to church was when I was seventeen," he shouted. "I have no interest in talking to you. Get out of here!" As the discomfited priest scuttled away, Charlie mumbled about his hatred for organized religion. Yet he had a strong faith in God. "Sure, I talk to God all the time, and I pray," he said. "I just don't need their rules and their priests to help me do it." He was certain he would meet God after he died.

For some people, neither their childhood religion nor any other traditional Western religion speaks to their spirituality. Many are influenced by Buddhism. Mr. Frank, a fifty-year-old patient who was dying of neck cancer, was one such person. He'd had a hard life. He grew up in a poor, inner-city home, facing the racism and poverty so common in the United States. In his twenties, he spent several years in prison for robbery. He took advantage of the prison's library to study several religions. He was impressed that, however different their theology, all shared a belief about the eternal nature of soul. His complete tranquillity in the face of his impending death was inspiring to all of us around him. He became a Buddhist and often spoke of how "we are soul in body, here to learn about life."

Others turn to New Age beliefs, which incorporate aspects of many ancient and modern belief systems. Marty was an elderly man dying of pancreatic cancer. He respected the Jewish religion he had grown up in, but it didn't move him in any spiritual way. He had married for a second time later in life, and his new wife had introduced him to the spiritual writings of Edgar Cayce and to the Foundation for Inner Peace book *A Course in Miracles* (Glen Ellen, CA, 1975). These works meant a lot to him, and he incorporated them into his own beliefs over the years. He approached his dying with great calm, seeing it in terms of what he called "the importance of pure love in our lives." He believed that such love was at the core of the universe, the true God, and he was confident that his death would simply be a return to that core.

A Few Suggestions

How can you discover your spiritual destiny? I have come up with a few suggestions, based on experiences I've had with patients. My suggestions may or may not work for you. You may find some useful and others not. They're meant less as a prescription than as a tool for coming up with your own method.

First of all, it may help to accept the idea, at least provisionally, that you have a spiritual destiny. Put aside your skepticism for a while: you can always reclaim it later. If you've gone through life without really thinking about the existence and importance of the spiritual nature of life, you might now find in your own mind a gentle tug, pulling you toward exploring some spiritual beliefs. Ask yourself if this is an area you want to continue exploring.

Second, you might want to ask questions about the role of spirituality in your own life to date. If you grew up in a religion, that may be a good starting place. Does it seem to you a truly spiritual religion? Does it answer some of your questions about a meaningful life? It may be that the *way* you were taught didn't offer much to you, but you can still search for something of value in it. Look deeper into the teachings of that religion. What do they say about the nature of living and dying?

If you don't find anything that resonates for you, continue your search by looking at other religions and spiritual teachings. At the core of virtually all religions is an attempt to answer the age-old questions about the meaning of life. You may find what works for you in one of these religions.

But you don't have to take on a specific religion. You may find that parts of many belief systems make sense for you, and you can use them as tools in developing your own core spirituality.

Perhaps none of the old teachings make sense for you. Seek further. Throughout the world, a spiritual awakening is taking place and many new interpretations of ancient core spirituality are taking form. This awakening includes the so-called New Age movement, but it is much larger and more diffuse.

The Question of Life after Death

At some point in my discussions with most people facing fatal illness, I often turn to the open-ended question of what happens to us after we die. Many of my patients find great peace in thinking that their soul will be united with some form of a higher power. But for some people, concern about payback for sins committed, continued suffering after dying, and fear of the unknown are stronger than any comfort their beliefs offer. People who have been raised in strict Christian religions often fear the eternal sufferings of hell. Among the patients I've worked with, however, I have seen more fear of purgatory than of hell. Perhaps this is because they have done the form of repentance their religion demands and feel secure that they won't suffer eternal damnation, but still believe that this leaves them with a residue of sin that must be purged with long-term pain. In such cases, I try to soothe their fears by further exploring why they believe their God will punish them. Often this helps them feel more hopeful about a peaceful meeting with a loving power after death.

One of my patients, Steve, was dying from advanced AIDS. At forty-five, he'd lived a troubled life, drifting from job to job and drinking a lot. His father had abandoned the family when Steve was a child; his mother had cared well for him in the years that followed, but he had never stopped mourning the loss of his father. He had grown into an angry, embittered man, driving everyone away with his hostility. In later years, he had begun to try to get his life together.

Now, lying in his hospital bed, unable to walk or even to feed himself, Steve asked to see me. He wanted to talk about his fears. "I'm going to spend a long time in purgatory," he told me.

I did not want to challenge the beliefs of his religion, but I did want to offer some reassurance. I spoke to him of my own belief: I could only imagine a loving God who would help him see the mistakes he had made in hurting others. I thought that this process would be positive and fair.

The next day, Steve told me he had thought over what I said and that the idea of a just and loving God made sense to him. He was able to move forward into his dying with greater peace, prepared to accept whatever the consequences of his actions would be, but with a sense that his purgatory might not be as harsh a place as he'd envisioned.

If you believe in and fear purgatory, you might be interested in reading the section of Dante's *Divine Comedy* known as *Purgatorio.* Everyone knows about the *Inferno,* this intensely religious medieval poet's portrait of the hideous sufferings of hell. But he sees purgatory very differently, as a place where suffering exists, but only to help the souls rid themselves of their earthly limitations. "Their sole motivation is charity, love of the supreme good," explains one Dante scholar. "Only, inasmuch as in their mortal lives there had been mixed in with this holy love, other loves, perverted or defective or excessive, in order to attain the perfect peace they must atone for these disordered loves." The penance, he adds, is the soul's own choice: it is cleansing itself for its return to God. Unlike the sufferings in the *Inferno,* those in the *Purgatorio* are suffused with joy and hope. I find this a far more reasonable vision of the transition into pure love, which is how Dante envisions *Paradiso.**

The belief in an afterlife can provide solace in a number of ways. It can help you look forward to being done with the pains of this life. If some of your loved ones have died, the hope of being reunited with them can be a great solace. It is a hope incorporated into the beliefs of most religions, and many people with no formal religion still have an understanding that the people they have loved will be with them in eternity. Certainly many of my own patients, coming from a variety of religious and spiritual beliefs, have anxiously looked forward to being with their lost parents, sons and daughters, spouses, and dear friends. Many

---

* Jefferson Butler Fletcher, *Dante* (Notre Dame, Ind.: University of Notre Dame Press, 1965), pp. 64–65; Paolo Milano, *The Portable Dante* (New York: Viking Press, 1947), pp. 267–268.

have said they knew they would be met by these people and ushered into their transition.

Near-Death Experiences

Sometimes, when it feels appropriate, I discuss with dying patients the interesting findings of near-death-experience researchers, such as Kenneth Ring (*Heading towards Omega*) and Ray Moody (*Life after Life*). These researchers, along with many others, have found that thousands of people, from different religions, countries, and cultures, have had astoundingly similar experiences. People describe being apart from their bodies, which they can see. Many hear a ringing or buzzing sound as they move rapidly through a tunnel. At the end of the tunnel is a bright blue or white light, and the spirits of relatives and friends who have died wait there. Details vary. Some people don't see the tunnel; some see Jesus or another religious figure waiting for them. But virtually all report experiencing an overwhelming feeling of love and peace before returning to their bodies.

I have come across similar experiences among my own patients. Many have come out of comas and described seeing the light, hearing the ringing sounds, and seeing loved ones awaiting them. Several dying people have told me that as they neared death, they felt a spark of eternal light, often blue or white, about to return them home to an ocean of light and love. One elderly patient had a particularly unusual vision. After coming out of a coma, he told me he had seen all the animals he had killed in his career as a rabbit farmer. He was strongly convinced that they had come to assure him that he was forgiven for his cruelty.

Such visions are somewhat rare, possibly because few people that close to death return to describe the experience. But most dying patients I've worked with have experienced being connected with a higher power and viewing illness and dying as a meaningful and significant part of living. This is truly discovering your spiritual destiny.

How all this works for you depends very much on what you believe. In my experience, most people do, as they die, feel in touch with a larger reality of which they are part. I know the cynical response to this—that it's simply desperate wishful thinking. Perhaps. But perhaps it's something much deeper—a capacity to see clearly for the first time, as the paraphernalia of daily living recedes from vision, what's really there.

CHAPTER 8

The Turning Point

❋ STEP L ❋
Being Ready

*I*T IS very possible that the treatments you're taking will either cure your disease or put you into long-term remission. But eventually, whether in the near future or years hence, the moment will come when you accept that you're dying. The process of dying often takes a lot of time, but most people, in their own way, know when they're closing in on the end. People with diseases like cancer often find it easier than some other patients to find this point of acceptance. Advancing heart, kidney, and lung disease often results in many episodes of severe illness, and sometimes it is difficult to decide when to stop fighting each episode with all your resources. Still, by heeding the progress of your illness, you can understand that you're ready to die. Recognizing that the end is approaching can be of enormous help to you, for now you're prepared to die—you're truly ready. This is the most profound turning point in your life. From this moment forward, it's important that you see dying as a natural and inevitable part of living, no longer as something to fight. Your job now is to let go of all material and emotional grasping and to begin to experience relaxation and closure in whatever way you can. The process of acceptance involves an appreciation of the quality of your life rather than the length of time it can be extended.

Discuss your feelings with your family and with your doctor. Your loved ones may have a lot of trouble with the fact that you're preparing to die. You are no longer denying death, but some of them still may be. You might find some of them quarreling with you, demanding that you change your mind and continue fighting to live. Let them know that what you need from them is support and love, not argument. They can't prevent your death, and they can only cause you pain by hanging on to you. Above all, make it clear to them that, whatever feelings they may have, your advance directives must at all times be honored.

When your loved ones accept your decision completely, they do both you and themselves a great service. Often at this time people find themselves transformed and released from barriers that have prevented them from expressing their love, forgiveness, and gratitude. You may find that you too are much more open to expressing such emotions than you were in the past. I have frequently worked with dying people who had never been very expressive, but who were able to transcend their reticence for a few moments to let their loved ones know how much they loved them.

Sometimes the communication doesn't happen in words. I watched the tender relationship between one of my dying patients and his fifty-year-old son. The younger man sat by his father's bedside every day for the last two weeks of the old man's life. I could never get them to speak to each other about their fears, but I soon realized I didn't have to. One day I sat with the two of them, and I spoke with them clearly about Mr. Diamond's imminent death. Both remained silent. But I saw Mr. Diamond look at his son as I spoke, and I knew that he was saying he was ready to die. His son looked back, his eyes saying that he understood and accepted this. The love these two silent men had for each other filled the room. I am still moved by the memory of that relationship and grateful that I was present to witness it.

In my experience, once people accept that they are ready to die, they are able to move along with the rest of their lives in a very natural, calm manner. It seems as if they will themselves to finish cleanly what needs to be finished and then to let go of this life. Often people are able to live long enough to experience a specific event—a wedding anniversary, a grandchild's gradua-tion—and then, the event completed, they die. This state of readiness gives you control over a very natural process. It makes dying a far less complicated process than it might otherwise be.

An oncologist colleague of mine describes the entrance to this phase beautifully. When it becomes clear to him that a pa-tient has reached a stage at which neither a cure nor a significant remission remains a realistic possibility, he tells the patient to ac-cept this and to follow the light. Peaceful dying is the only rea-sonable goal at this point.

Reaching this level of readiness allows you to arrange all your affairs and be certain that everything you want to say is said, everything you want to do is done. This is an opportunity that those who die suddenly never get to experience, and you are blessed to have it.

⋆ STEP M ⋆
Shifting to Care

Once you are ready, palliative care—care geared toward relieving suffering and helping the patient die comfortably and peacefully, rather than toward cure—is your most important priority. All acute cure-based medical treatment must stop. Measures meant to cure disease are no longer appropriate and, indeed, are likely to interfere with the palliative care you now need. It is important for your doctors, family, and friends to respect your decision to focus on palliative care as much as they did your earlier efforts at cure. The medical staff and your family must honor your choice and attempt to ensure that your wishes be fulfilled at every step in the process.

If you are suffering from worsening heart, lung, kidney, or infectious disease, you may wish to use both curative intervention and palliative care. The curative measures are often those that relieve discomfort. The difference between curative and palliative care isn't always clear, and you may need to balance the two. Once you have passed the Being Ready stage, your emphasis is on the palliative, rather than the curative, aspects of care.

However, just as you face the possibility of resistance from your family, you may also face it from your doctors and nurses. The current medical system continues to have great difficulty in shifting from attempts to cure disease and prevent death to treatment plans that focus on providing comfort-based care. Keep in mind that doctors still are usually not well trained in the physical, psychological, and spiritual techniques of providing comfort care to the dying. Because medical schools offer little psychological training in this area, the chances are strong that many of your health care workers will not be comfortable with providing comfort care. (The major exception is palliative-care clinicians; see Chapter 9, Step Q.) You may feel some anger toward your medical workers, but try to contain it and instead talk with them about your wishes and firmly insist that they respect these wishes.

Throughout years of working in hospitals and clinics, I have heard doctors and nurses discuss advanced illness with patients and say, petulantly, "Well, if you don't do anything, you'll just die." Of course you will. You'll "just die" even if you continue with cure-based treatments. Despite all our efforts and medical intervention, we are all going to die at some point.

Once you've decided to shift from medical treatments aimed at curing disease to comfort care, you need to know that your doctors won't abandon you as a patient and that you will be protected from unnecessary pain. You have the right to ask for your doctor's reassurance. If the response is, "There's nothing more I can do for you," challenge that. Medicine can still help you achieve your goal. The doctor who has tried to cure you now should shift to helping you die peacefully.

If the doubts of your loved ones or your doctors make you nervous, don't worry. You'll always have the option as time progresses to switch back and forth, balancing cure-based and care-based treatment. It may be helpful to speak to a hospital-based social worker or a claims representative from your insurance company to define clearly what your insurance covers. You may ask a family member to check on the length of stay that your Medicare benefits cover as well as on other insurance allotments. It's always helpful to know what benefits you can expect when you're making health care decisions. In this age of increased managed care, some of the most comprehensive end-of-life programs are going to be found within HMOs.

❧ STEP N ❧
Ensuring Family Support

Having decided on comfort care, you must be assured that your wishes for this specific kind of care will be carried out. Your loved ones will be able to help you request and obtain the kind of care you want. Once you stop requesting cure-based treatment, your doctor may have less and less to offer you. Insist, and have your family and friends insist on your behalf, that you get the best palliative care your area has to offer.

Such care will be available in varying degrees in different parts of the country. In general, you're more likely to find expertise in palliative care in a hospice—a facility designed specifically to treat people who have fewer than six months to live—or at home with the help of hospice workers (see Chapter 9, Step Q).

Since hospitals are geared toward acute medicine rather than palliative care, your hospital staff may not be as knowledgeable as you might wish about palliative care. If you'll be dying in a hospital, it's important to make sure that the hospital you choose has a skilled practitioner on staff who is experienced in pain management and end-of-life care, or has access to such an expert. It's a good idea to have another family meeting in which the family listens to your specific requests. Your decision for comfort care means that you have faced your advancing illness with strength, dignity, and courage. Your loved ones can now help you carry out your wishes. In the near future, you and your loved ones will need to decide where you want to die. This is a great opportunity to increase your closeness and camaraderie with your loved ones.

Sometimes you need to communicate to people who might be hesitant to visit you for a number of reasons. As noted in Chapter 4, people are sometimes reluctant to face dying loved ones because it challenges their own denial of mortality. When they do visit, they may do so only briefly, talk incessantly to avoid facing what's happening to you, or have stopped off at a bar first. Such visits may not be pleasant for you, and you might want to keep them brief. You have a right to guard your privacy, and that includes restricting visits that are too stressful to enjoy. You can also ask these people to come at certain times and not when they've been drinking.

Further, there are always people who are convinced that they'll catch your disease from you. This happens not only with contagious diseases like AIDS, but even with noncommunicable diseases like cancer. Such people need to have a solid conversation with a patient medical professional who can clarify that they can't get AIDS from hanging out with someone and they can't catch cancer from someone no matter *what* they're doing together.

Children who have been important in your life should also

be brought to see you. Our society has a tendency to shield children from death and dying, making it far more fearsome than it need be. No matter how young children are, they can benefit from visiting with loved ones. Few children are frightened when they visit the bedside of someone who's dying, unless the adults around them show fear. Visits with the children in your life can be wonderfully comforting to you and can also help the children understand the naturalness of death.

You'll also want to be certain that your health care proxy and all your loved ones fully understand your instructions. You may need certain kinds of medical equipment, or particular foods, and you want to be assured that your needs will be met right up until your death. You'll want to be assured that when you can no longer speak, your proxy will say just what you want said to your doctors, family members, and other important people. Finally, you'll want to know that your entire medical team understands and agrees to honor your advance request not to prolong your life by technical means.

It's important that you get all of these assurances long before you become too weak to understand, or slip into a coma. Make certain that no one who can't honor your decisions has any power over you when you no longer have power over yourself.

✦ STEP O ✦
Talking to Your Doctor Again

It's important now that you talk with your doctor to make sure that your doctor fully understands your decision. Medical care in hospitals runs on doctors' orders; if your doctor's orders don't match your wishes, the orders will still be followed. Your family can advocate for you, but even family members can be overruled by the doctor. If you haven't done so already, you might at this point want to add a do-not-resuscitate request to your living will (see Chapter 6, Step I). If you do, be sure to discuss it with your doctor. You'll probably have to be the one to initiate the conversation; doctors rarely do. Explain that you want everything possible done to keep you comfortable, but you don't want your life prolonged with any technology. Make sure your doctors agree with your decision.

You may be uncomfortable asking your doctor to follow your wishes, but you have to overcome your embarrassment. If you don't, the lack of communication may result in your getting treatments you don't want. You can't afford any ambiguity around this issue. I've seen many doctor-patient relationships suffer terribly because this kind of frank conversation never took place. Remember that you and your doctor are in partnership around your caretaking, and this kind of partnership requires honesty and clarity.

You may feel it is unfair that you have to take the initiative. In an ideal world, you wouldn't. But until medical schools and residency programs train doctors in all aspects of caring for the dying, this responsibility will probably fall on patients and their families. Perhaps it may help to realize that in this area, *you* are the expert. What you teach your doctor in the process of clarifying your own needs and wishes may help that doctor in dealing with future patients.

✦ STEP P ✦
Dealing with the Suicide Question

In the past few years suicide has been a hot topic and Kevorkian a household name. Indeed, it seems as though in the perception of much of the public the chief route to peaceful dying is doctor-assisted suicide. I find this tragic. While I wouldn't quarrel with anyone's right to choose suicide, I don't think it's ever the best decision. And the main reasons people do choose suicide stem from predictable and preventable circumstances. One reason is the fear of pain. Advocates for physician-assisted suicide suggest that it is the way to avoid the terrible pain that many dying people experience in the last days and weeks of their lives. But suicide isn't the only solution to that problem. It can seem that way, but it wouldn't if good end-of-life caretaking were available. As I'll discuss in the next chapter, excellent pain-relief drugs exist that can help virtually all dying patients.

The other major reason people who are dying choose suicide is that they fear the loss of control that usually accompanies dying—the total inability to care for themselves. Suicide certainly is a means of taking control of your life and your death. But, as I will illustrate shortly, there are other ways to control the events of your dying days and also ways to accept the loss of control as part of the natural rhythm of life.

Suicide as an end-of-life alternative, particularly when it's physician assisted, makes me uncomfortable for a number of reasons. For one thing, the idea of doctors, trained to heal, becoming professional killers isn't a very attractive one. It's a privilege for a doctor to help a patient face the last days of life with dignity and comfort and to participate in the amazing emotional and spiritual growth that so often accompanies a measured dying. But to actually bring about death—that's something else.

I am also concerned about what it means to society when we accept doctors' killing patients, even with the most benevolent of intentions. How often is the request for suicide fueled by clinical, and treatable, depression? How far a step from this is it to killing people who haven't asked to die? Many people with advanced illnesses can't make their wishes known, because of dementia conditions such as Alzheimer's or because their illnesses have created paralysis. Perhaps some of these people are inconvenient to their families, or the nursing homes where they live, or the hospital staffs. I know that in the Netherlands, where doctor-assisted suicide is not illegal, there are controls, and presumably there would be in the United States as well, but it's an awfully dangerous door to open. At present, we have no standardized counselng for the dying. How can we wisely introduce physician-assisted suicide without a comprehensive model of evaluating and counseling about the emotions that cause a patient to request assisted suicide?

Cecily Saunders, the powerful woman credited with starting the modern hospice movement in the United Kingdom, addressed assisted suicide by stating, "Those most experienced in meeting the difficult medical, nursing, and above all, personal and social problems that are now referred to hospice teams are the very people who see the most compelling arguments against euthanasia, understood as the deliberate shortening of life. We know something of the potentials in treatment, and are learning all the time, and we believe in personal growth, even to the end of life, however diminished it may look."*

Some of my colleagues have suggested that, while it may be wrong for a doctor to actually do the killing, it's less problematic to simply supply the means of suicide to a patient who asks for it. At least, they argue, an overdose of barbiturates would be less painful and less chancy than other methods the patient might choose. But again, this involves a healer in killing. I can't judge the morality of other doctors, but I know that I could never supply the means of suicide to a patient. It seems to me far more useful for a doctor to ask why the patient is considering suicide and then try to address those concerns in other ways.

When I work with dying patients, I always ask what their fears about dying are. When patients are thinking about suicide, I also ask why they think suicide would be a better route than

---

* Cecily Saunders, *Death without Dignity: Euthanasia in Perspective* (Edinburgh: Rutherford House, 1990), p. 92.

seeing the experience out. Most respond that they are terribly afraid of uncontrolled pain, of humiliation from their body's deteriorating, of causing their loved ones to suffer, and of losing control over their lives. When we examine in depth each of these fears, as we will in the next chapter, a solution to each usually becomes clear.

Unfortunately, most communities don't offer trained counselors who can help dying people work through these fears. During my medical training I saw scores of patients lying alone in their hospital beds, terrified of their impending deaths, with no one to talk to. Is it any wonder that to avoid facing this prospect, so many people contemplate suicide?

Thinking about suicide can actually be healthy for a dying patient. You've been dealt a terrible blow; you're frightened; and you're probably angry at fate or at God or at all the doctors who haven't been able to make you well again. The process of contemplating suicide and what it means to you can be a major part of the growing that takes place during your dying months.

It's interesting to me to see how few dying patients really do kill themselves, even in countries where physician-assisted suicide is readily available. The possibility is always there, yet only a handful seize it. Most of the patients I've worked with have talked about suicide from time to time, but only one has ever chosen to do it, swallowing a handful of pills in order to prevent further suffering from his stomach cancer. He killed himself early in his contact with his health care team. I believe that he had not had enough support and counseling. His depression and his refusal to look at lifelong issues made it very hard for anyone on the staff to reach him.

I think that in the future more and more patients will demand counseling specifically dealing with the question of suicide, whether on one's own or assisted by a doctor, and that increasingly fewer will choose suicide.

For those who are truly determined to commit suicide, I would respect and honor their right to make that choice. But I could never be a participant in the process or provide the means to make it possible. I realize that this isn't always a popular position. Many people disagree with me: my coauthor feels strongly that suicide is a reasonable option, as do some of my closest friends. I respect their views, but I don't agree with them.

It might be helpful to you to try to understand your own doctor's views on physician-assisted suicide. When you feel comfortable, you can ask about these views directly. What you learn may or may not affect your own decision.

Part of my own outlook is a deeply held philosophical belief—or perhaps I should say spiritual belief. I don't accept the view of those religions that say a person who commits suicide will suffer for all eternity. That cruel and unforgiving God is alien to me, though he certainly has been very real for some of the patients I have worked with. But I think that belief may originate in an important truth—a recognition of the fundamental unnaturalness of suicide. It seems to me that we were given this life to experience some things and learn some things, and that suicide cuts off the possibility of doing that fully. I believe that we are connected to a greater whole and that dying is a part of living that should not be altered to suit our perceptions, especially if we want to experience this sense of connectedness.

Several of my patients have shared my feelings about suicide, though often coming from a different perspective. One of them expressed his thoughts beautifully to me. Ed, sixty-two years old, had a terrible tumor in the back of his mouth, so huge that he could no longer eat and was getting his nutrition from a gastric tube. Several years earlier, he'd become involved with the Rosicrucian religion, which includes a belief in reincarnation. It was hard for him to talk because of the tumor, which was invading his neck and making his voice very soft, but he talked anyway.

He had considered suicide—he was in a great deal of discomfort—but discarded it. "If I kill myself, I'll just have to come back in my next life into the same kind of situation I'm in now, and I'll have to learn all this stuff again. If I go through dying, my soul will be free at the end of this, and it will move on to wherever it has to go." He used his dying weeks to become reunited with his estranged son and his four-year-old grandson.

The question of suicide came closer to home for me several years ago when my father-in-law was diagnosed with metastatic esophageal cancer. He called and asked me to get him a lethal dose of barbiturates, which had been described in the Hemlock Society's literature. I was horrified, but I tried to stay calm. I realized that he had always prided himself on his control and that suicide seemed to him the best way to retain that control. He knew what the last days of life could be like and didn't want to be helpless, unable to control his bladder and bowels. "I think you want your family to remember your dying with grace," I told him, "but suicide might not be the best way to create that. I promise you that I can help you to truly die with grace."

My father-in-law and I talked for a long while. The more he thought about it, the more he realized that he could handle the dying process. He decided to die at home, and we worked out a good caretaking schedule. His wife was able to be his primary caregiver, and together with the local home-based hospice support (see Chapter 9, Step Q), they worked out the details. When it became necessary, a hospital bed was brought to his room. Gradually, naturally, his mind and body slowed down. He had time to be with his grandchildren and his five grown children. My wife and I lived in a different state, but we went to see him frequently. I vividly recall my last visit with him, several weeks before he died. His eyes were very bright, his head large compared to his frail, skin-and-bones body. But he was happy. His last few days were all he had feared—he was totally weakened, unable to leave his bed, and incontinent—yet the fear and repugnance were gone. He was totally at peace. He slipped into a coma and died painlessly. His struggle with the question of suicide and the way he lived out his last days were among the richest experiences I have witnessed.

If you are considering killing yourself, I'd ask you to look deeply into your reasons. I am convinced that very few dying people would choose to end their own lives if they had confidence that they had decent alternatives. There *are* such alternatives, as I discuss elsewhere in this book.

I've heard some people speak of suicide as a means of saving their loved ones from pain. This is truly self-defeating. The knowledge of a loved one's suicide, especially if it hasn't been discussed beforehand, can be a terrible burden for the survivor. At the very least, think it through thoroughly. Make sure you've given yourself every opportunity to consider all the other possible paths. Perhaps after doing so, you'll still think about taking your own life. But I truly doubt it.

CHAPTER 9

Preventing Pain and Isolation

✳ STEP Q ✦
Deciding Where to Die

O NE OF the most important decisions you can make at this time is whether to approach your dying at home or in an institution. Approximately 80 percent of the U.S. population die in a hospital or nursing home, and 20 percent choose to stay at home or to die in a hospice inn.

Dying at Home

When it's possible, dying at home—your own home or that of a loved one—is probably the best alternative. It provides many advantages over institutionalized dying, and indeed more and more people are making this choice. Dying at home allows you to be in familiar and comfortable surroundings, without the regimens and sterility of a hospital setting. It also gives you the largest degree of control over your own dying process. For these reasons, it's wise to consider this option seriously. Most patients I've worked with have preferred to die at home when their circumstances permitted it.

To make dying at home work, someone must become the primary caregiver responsible for coordinating all your activities. Usually this caregiver is a capable, mature family member or loved one who is willing to take on this responsibility and service. But even if you have someone who is able to stay home and take care of you full-time, this isn't a one-person job. The primary caregiver must have the support of a hired or voluntary aide, as well as some training from a skilled health practitioner. Sometimes, families and friends are able to share the primary job so that the primary caregiver isn't just one person.

It can be very helpful for you and your caregiver to enlist the aid of a hospice program. These programs do an excellent job of providing the assistance necessary to enable families to keep their loved ones at home. Members of the hospice team include nurses, social workers, home health aides, and volunteers. Some of these people will come to your home, evaluate your requirements, and walk you and your caregiver through this difficult and important time of life.

Most likely you will need guidance with issues ranging from how to get a hospital bed into the house to addressing such caregiving needs as home oxygen, commodes, disposable bedding, bandages, wheelchairs, and walkers. Hospice workers can also answer questions caregivers may have, such as, Is it legal to allow someone to die at home? How will we deal with shortness of breath, increasing pain, and bowel problems? What do we do with the body once the person has died? Make certain that you and your caregivers make lists of all your questions in advance.

Equally important, your caregiver will need emotional and practical help through the transition of bringing you from the hospital to the home. It also makes sense to coordinate the decision to stay at home with your primary medical doctor, cleric, and any other personal support systems.

Many people have fears about caring for someone who is dying at home. If this is the case with your loved ones, it may be easier to hire a nurse to take care of you, if you can afford to do so.

Caring for a loved one at home allows family members,

friends, and even pets to move about without the restrictions of an institutional setting. People can cook you special meals, make sure you have your favorite objects around you, and do all the little things that create a cozy, pleasant atmosphere for you. And if enough of your close friends and family members live nearby, you can be sure of having some of the people you care most about with you all the time. Many dying people are afraid of being alone in the days and weeks preceding their actual dying. Being at home can help you with the disorientation that frequently occurs at night in unfamiliar hospital surroundings.

Being home also allows you the most flexibility. There are no rules about numbers of visitors or visiting hours, no restrictions on what you can or can't do. So you can, with your caregiver's help, control most aspects of your dying.

A wonderful story illustrates this point. An acquaintance of mine had a friend who ran a jazz club in New Orleans. He loved jazz passionately, and many of his friends were jazz musicians. While he was dying, he decided that it was silly to have his wake when he couldn't be there to enjoy it—so he had his wake at home. It was a huge, round-the-clock party: artists and musicians flew from around the world to join it. There was food, drink, and above all, music—a giant farewell blast.

A raucous party may not be your style, but you can create the environment and the rituals of your own dying. You can make of your dying not just a departure from your life, but a celebration of it.

The process of dying will involve degrees of suffering for you, and your primary caregiver will need everyone's support. It's important that nobody panic when your bodily functions slow down: all your physical changes can be handled at home with the proper support. There is no reason for you to end up in the hospital getting acute care when you truly want to stay at home and die there. Trained hospice workers or home health aides can give your caregiver specific recommendations for dealing with breathing difficulties, digestive problems, incontinence, bed sores, pain control, and emotional agitation. And if you're working with hospice help or other home health care aides, doctors and nurses will be available for phone consultations twenty-four hours a day.

Although dying at home is often the best way to achieve a peaceful process, it isn't the right decision for everyone. Dying at home can be expensive, since insurance companies pay for only some home health care (though this may be changing soon, as more insurance companies come to realize that palliative care is less costly than traditional hospital care). Either a full-time home health aide has to be hired, or one of your caregivers needs to stay at home rather than work at an outside job. Much depends on how large, and how available, your caregiving network is.

If you are considering dying at home, you and your caregivers must take several factors into consideration. The first and most basic question is whether there is a primary caregiver who can do the job. This role can be very rewarding; it is a great act of love that can mean as much to the caregiver as to the person being cared for. I have spoken with many people who have taken on this responsibility and have found that they have never regretted the time and effort put into the care of a dying person who was important to them.

Like most deeply rewarding tasks, however, being a dying person's primary caregiver isn't easy. Your caregiver can get assistance from family members and friends, home health care aides, hospice volunteers, and neighbors, but this person will have the greatest responsibility and in all likelihood the greatest amount of work to do for you. Often people assume that a full-time homemaker can easily absorb one more responsibility in the home, but this isn't necessarily true. Raising children, even teenagers, can be a twenty-four-hour-a-day job that leaves little room for added responsibility. Sometimes, a person may be able to give up a full-time job to care for a loved one at home, but this is not always feasible.

Your primary caregiver—or caregivers (in many cases, friends and family members share the primary job)—must be physically strong enough to help you as you become less mobile and emotionally strong enough to handle the daily, intimate tasks associated with the dying process, such as changing diapers. And your caregiver needs to have a lot of patience: as you grow weaker, your demands will inevitably become greater.

Once you've chosen your primary caregiver, you need to discuss what the responsibilities are and what backup will be in place. It would be wise to meet with all your friends and family members who will be part of the caretaking network and arrange as far as possible specific responsibilities and time commitments. All your caregivers, not only the primary one, need to be clear about what their responsibilities are and commit only to what they can reasonably expect of themselves.

Your caregivers also need to give thought to what they will do when you are actually dying. The sights and sounds can be frightening to someone who isn't prepared. Suddenly your breathing is going, and the caregiver seems to become completely incompetent—it can feel like an emergency, and the caregiver's impulse may be to dial 911. This is a perfectly good impulse in a situation involving a healthy person or one assumed to be capable of recovery. But if you're dying and have chosen to do so without intervention, your caregiver shouldn't call 911. You don't want to be rushed to the hospital, attached to all kinds of machines, and die precisely the way you've chosen *not* to die. Your caregivers will need guidance beforehand about how to handle this crucial moment.

Further, while having someone you love become your caregiver can deepen the bonds between you, it can in some cases weaken them. I know of one case in which a woman quit her job to take care of her mother, but the strain of the mother's dying and the daughter's feeling of sacrifice created bickering, guilt, and anger. "Our relationship deteriorated badly," the younger woman said later. "If I had kept my job and just visited her a lot, we both would have been better off." People need to respect their own limits, and not feel guilty for doing only what they can for you within these limits. Nor should you feel unloved or abandoned if no one is able to provide the structure for your home care. I've seen much love and much resolution take place in ordinary hospital rooms.

In this short discussion, I have been able only to touch on the issue of dying at home. If you are considering this choice, I recommend that you and your loved ones read Andrea Sankar's *Dying at Home: A Family Guide for Caregiving* (see Appendix 4). It is an excellent and thorough exploration of the decision in every aspect.

Dying in the Hospital

Most people dread the idea of dying in a hospital, and with reason. Hospitals tend to be impersonal, uncomfortable, and rigid. A hospital is structured to be run as a paramilitary system. The food is standardized and often tasteless; the decor is stark, and the lighting awful. None of this matters too much if you're in there for a relatively brief time: you have your surgery, you recover, and in a few days you leave for the comfort of your own home. But it's not a structure well suited for a peaceful dying.

A hospital does have advantages, however. You get twenty-four-hour-a-day professional care, allowing your loved ones to spend as much time as they can with you while continuing to live their own lives and meet all their responsibilities.

Most hospitals are beginning to change their approach to

caring for the dying. With the ascendancy of managed care, which insists on shortened stays, hospitals are finding that they have a lot of empty beds. So more and more of them are turning over rooms to what they call hospice care. This is comfort-care oriented, not acute-care oriented. You can choose inpatient hospice care if your local hospital has this service. Many communities have an inpatient hospice available either freestanding or within a hospital facility. You can call your local hospital or local hospice group to refer you to an inpatient hospice.

Inpatient hospice rooms are usually more attractive than traditional hospital rooms. They're intended as places in which people will live out their last days, rather than as temporary stops for people who will be treated for acute problems and then released. The rooms are pleasantly decorated, with carpeting, plants, attractive wall hangings, and soft lighting. This is a big step forward, but it's not enough.

The problem is that by and large, hospitals are just beginning to train their staffs in how to care properly for the dying. Often staff from the main floor are given brief, on-the-job guidelines, but not the in-depth training necessary to make a big difference. They loosen up on the rigidity of visiting hours so that your friends and family can come see you, but they often don't offer counseling to help your loved ones deal with their own feelings and relate to you in the best way. Few hospitals have social workers or doctors trained to facilitate the kinds of meetings with friends and family discussed in Chapter 5, and few have doctors who are fully trained in palliative care.

However, if you're spending your last days in such a setting, don't despair: you're not helpless. You and your loved ones can take steps to make the experience close to what you need. I'll address pain relief later in this chapter: it exists, and you can fight for access to it. You can also ask that someone trained in family counseling meet with you and your loved ones. Hospice rooms are a new concept for hospitals, and in demanding what you need, you'll help define what they can become. Further, such rooms do offer you the space to live out your remaining life in comfort and, if you choose, to do the spiritual work discussed in Chapter 7.

You can create a comfortable environment for your dying even in a regular hospital room. Your loved ones can bring things you need for emotional comfort—your favorite quilt, photos of people you love, the kinds of things that create an ambiance of home.

Rooms in hospitals, whether hospice rooms or regular rooms, can be private or semiprivate. Sometimes sharing a room is great. If you and your roommate have a lot in common, or hit it off well, you can be excellent company for each other. You can laugh, share stories, and keep loneliness at bay when your family and friends aren't around.

On the other hand, a roommate can be a problem if you need solitude. One patient I worked with was so desperate for solitude that he made his covers into a tent and spent most of his time inside it. Eventually, he was transferred to a private room.

Even if you are gregarious, it can be difficult having a roommate who is at a different stage of illness. If you're feeling fairly well and expect to be around a little longer, it can be hard to share a room with someone in the last stages of dying. As I discuss in Step S, Dealing with Physical Changes, usually the process of dying involves unpleasant sights and odors, which can be disturbing. At the same time, you might be the sole companion of a dying roommate and can help comfort that person, which can bring comfort to you as well.

Depending on how strong you are, you may be able to leave the hospital for brief times. Your friends and family should remember that. It might be very important to you to be present at weddings, graduations, and other events in the lives of those you love. One of the patients I worked with asked to go home for an afternoon simply to eat a sandwich under his favorite tree in his backyard.

Ask for the people closest to you to be more than just visitors. In *Dying at Home,* Andrea Sankar describes how people train themselves for caregiving in the home by beginning when the dying person is still in the hospital. Her descriptions apply equally to this situation: "A caretaker who actively participates in the care of a hospitalized patient has far more opportunity to observe the patient's condition and response to different medications than the professionals involved in that care. These observations can provide valuable information for professionals in their attempts to relieve the patient's distress and maintain comfort."* Such caregivers, Sankar adds, can also help make sure that doctors are doing what the patient wants and that the staff follows the doctors' orders. Busy nurses, she points out, often can't provide the amount of attention the dying person needs, and friends and family can fill in the gaps. This kind of caregiving can be a great privilege for the people who love you. They may not have the resources to do full-time caretaking in a home environment, but they may still want to contribute some time and energy to your well-being.

If you are dying in a hospital, you may want to pay attention to the importance of developing a good relationship with your nursing staff. Nurses are well-trained professionals who are usually extremely skilled at meeting the physical and emotional needs of individual patients. Nursing and nursing education have always focused on treating the whole patient—body, mind, and spirit. You'll find most nurses very open to discussing your joys and fears with you. Talk honestly with your nurses and nurs-

---

* Andrea Sankar, *Dying at Home: A Family Guide for Caregiving* (New York: Bantam Books, 1998), pp. 17–25.

ing assistants—you're likely to find that you're greatly helped by their experience and knowledge.

VISITORS

There are other people you'll want to see, people who may not have the inclination or ability to be caregivers, but are still people you care about and enjoy seeing. Visits with friends are an important part of living, and they can be an important part of the dying process.

Most hospitals will bend the rules limiting the number of visitors, especially to a hospice unit. But if yours doesn't, you can find creative ways to see everyone you want. If several people come at once, some can wait outside the room and you can rotate visitors. The important thing is to create the best environment for yourself in whatever ways are possible.

If you have pets, your family and friends should be allowed to bring them to visit you. People often have very deep relationships with animals, and being separated from pets can be a real loss. You may have to arrange for specific times for animal visits, but most hospitals with hospice rooms will have some such visiting hours.

CREATURE COMFORT

Never dismiss the importance of supposedly minor needs. One of the most important people in an inpatient hospice is the hairdresser. It's amazing how invigorated patients can feel after having their hair done. Most hospitals don't have resident hairdressers, but you can ask your friends and family to search for one who will visit the hospital. Don't hesitate to make these kinds of demands if you think they'll make a difference to you.

You'll probably want to avoid using hospital sheets and nightclothes—they're dreary, sterile, and institutional. Instead, bring—or have your family bring—your own sheets, blankets, nightgowns or pajamas, robes, and slippers. Bring a lamp so you don't have to rely on the hospital's overhead lighting: you want soft, comfortable lighting. If possible, avoid harsh fluorescent lighting. Bring your TV and VCR, along with your favorite tapes, so you can watch the TV shows and movies you most enjoy. Bring lots of books; surround yourself with your favorite authors. The hospital bed is probably your last home; it should be as comfortable as any home you've ever lived in.

One thing that can contribute to your comfort is physical touch. You're still living in your body, and it still needs attention. Having a good massage therapist come to the hospital can be a great help. Many hospitals have nurses trained in massage therapy.

RITUALS

Rituals are important in every aspect of living, and they are often even more important in dying. These can be small, domestic rituals, such as drinking your orange juice from a particular glass. They can be traditional celebrations of holidays and birthdays. Spiritual rituals are often very healing. They can be as simple as having a few loved ones pray with you or they can be more complex. One patient I recall from my early training was Mr. Avon, a Native American in his forties who was dying of lymphoma. His dying involved rituals from his tradition. He was never left alone: people from his family and members of his spiritual group sat with him all the time. They held a vigil for two weeks before he died. One of these people was a shaman, his friend, who helped him organize his rituals. Mr. Avon had a private room, which was important for him since his rituals involved burning incense. It was crucial to his spiritual practice that no one come into his room without taking his or her shoes off. I enjoyed watching the startled expressions on the faces of doctors and nurses when they were asked, politely but firmly, to take off their shoes. To their credit, none of them ever protested.

Not all rituals are possible in every setting, however. Lighting candles or incense can cause problems if there's oxygen in the room—you could blow the place up. Some hospitals won't permit lighting candles because of the possibility of fire. Nonetheless, the staff often allow a patient to bend the rules a little. When my coauthor's brother was dying, she wanted to do a spiritual ritual with him that involved burning candles. The nurse told her that would set off the fire alarm, but, she added, it would take a few minutes for this to happen. Would it be enough to burn the candle for only a minute or so? It was, and my coauthor and her brother were able to continue their ritual.

Incense can cause problems if you are sharing a room. The smell might appeal to your roommate, but it also might trigger allergic reactions or nausea. You need to negotiate with whoever has a problem with what you're doing and try to reach a creative compromise. Perhaps you can burn the incense just long enough for you to smell it, but not long enough for it to permeate the room. Perhaps you can gain some of the benefits by simply having the candle or the incense with you.

More and more, the effectiveness of healing techniques once dismissed by Western medicine is being recognized, and I think this recognition will continue to grow as we see these techniques work. At this point in your life, you're not looking for the cure aspect of these traditions, but for the comfort aspect—an equally significant part of healing.

I always remember with glee the room of one of my patients, a big, burly, tattooed man from the Catskill mountain area. He did everything. There were nurses doing Therapeutic Touch, psychic healers, Reiki healers—every conceivable alternative healer. He had candles and incense—he was very well armed. It was invigorating to enter his room: people felt good when they walked into its cheerful, lively atmosphere. He knew he was dying: this wasn't a desperate effort to be cured. He wanted to die comfortably, and he was making that happen. It was very unlike the rooms in which visitors were looking depressed and upset. Here, everyone felt part of an authentic healing process.

Nursing Homes

Increasingly, older people are dying not in a hospital but in a nursing home. Many of the same issues apply to both. Usually in a nursing home you'll have no trouble decorating your room (or your half of a shared room) as you please, since these rooms are designed for living, not for acute medical care. If you're in a nursing home, it's important to make certain that your advance directives include your wishes about hospitalization. For example, if you want to die in the nursing home, you don't want an emergency transfer to a hospital in the middle of the night. The decision can be complicated, so you'll want to think it through thoroughly. Will you want to be hospitalized if you develop pneumonia? For someone who is dying, pneumonia can often be a blessing—the body closes down before more difficult symptoms bring on death. On the other hand, pneumonia might cut short a few weeks that are precious to you. Similarly, you'll want your wishes about feeding tubes specified. It's important to have these desires written down formally and to discuss them with your family as early as possible in case you become physically unable to speak for yourself (see Chapter 6, Step I).

Hospice Inns

Hospice care is based on a philosophy of comfort care for the dying, rather than the hospital approach of drastic interventions. The hospice movement usually works with people who are dying at home, but there are a number of hospice inns in the United States. These inns take only patients whose doctors have given them a prognosis of six months or less to live, so you won't have access to a hospice if you have been given a longer prognosis.

If you decide you want to die in a hospice inn, you should start looking into it as early on as possible. Talk to your doctor: some hospices accept only people who have been referred by physicians. Sadly, many doctors remain unwilling to make such referrals. Too many are suspicious of the hospice movement; they feel they can take care of their patients perfectly well. You need to be polite with such doctors. Remind them that they're busy and can't be there as often as you'd like for pain consultations and other questions and that you really don't want to spend your last days in a hospital environment. You can find a hospice near you by calling your local hospital or one of the resource numbers listed in Appendix 4 for information.

✻ STEP R ✻
Getting Relief for Your Pain

Excellent pain control and constant reevaluation of your physical comfort are available—and they are essential. There are many ways to control pain adequately, and there is never an acceptable reason for a doctor to ignore your complaint of pain.

Numerous studies and clinical teachings have shown the importance of balancing narcotic and nonnarcotic pain medicine to keep a dying person comfortable and alert. Certain narcotic medications are highly effective in controlling the pain from advanced cancers, and I've seen many patients remain lucid and comfortable on high doses. Arguments for not using narcotics to ease pain because they may cause addiction are biased and outdated: at this point in your life, you're not likely to start robbing liquor stores to get your fix. Unfortunately, modern medical education has still not adequately emphasized teaching pain control, especially in caring for the dying. Therefore, many doctors are uncomfortable with this aspect of delivering health care and too many people suffer from intense pain when they are dying. It's extremely important that you discuss this aspect of care with your primary physician as early as possible.

Your family members and loved ones may need to demand additional medical and pharmacological consultations if your pain is not being managed adequately. It may take several requests to persuade your primary and consulting physicians that whenever you complain of pain, you should immediately be given the appropriate medication. The importance of pain management has always been obvious to the nursing profession. As palliative comfort care becomes integrated into mainstream health care delivery, doctors will increasingly come to recognize its importance. A number of educational programs are being developed within the medical community to increase physicians' knowledge and experience with pain management.

If your own doctor isn't able to relieve your pain, demand a consultation with one who can. Every community has a palliative care physician or a clinical pharmacologist. If necessary, get your family or friends to do some research. Find out who the nearby experts in pain management are and then insist on a consultation with one or more of those experts. Almost all pain can be alleviated with a combination of medicines, and there is no excuse for your doctor not to work at solving a difficult case. For the rare situation in which the pain doesn't respond to the pain-control drugs, it can be relieved with a combination of these drugs and strong sedatives.

In this computer age, pain-control experts are more accessible than they were in the past. If no one can come to you, you can use telecommunications. Tell your doctor, nurse, or social worker to phone the expert, explain what medications you're on, and get advice.

In this area, too, your friends and family can be of enormous help to you. If you're not getting through to your doctors, get your loved ones to help you in your fight by politely reinforcing your demands. You should never have to be in pain, and requests for pain medication should never go unanswered.

⇥ STEP S ⇤
Dealing with Physical Changes

Dying brings about dramatic physical changes that you and your caregivers must anticipate.

Loss of Appetite and Thirst

The first significant change is the slowing of bodily functions, which naturally causes a decrease in appetite. As I noted in Chapter 6, Step I, you have to let go of everything you take for granted about food, eating, and keeping up your strength. You won't starve to death. There will be no pain associated with the loss of appetite. In the later stages of slowing down you may want only liquids and very small food portions. Similarly, you'll probably experience a gradual loss of thirst. At times you'll need only a few ice chips to moisten and soothe your mouth and lips.

The diminished need for food and drink is part of the body's natural preparation to stop functioning. You shouldn't be forced or even encouraged to eat if you don't want to. This is sometimes a difficult concept for family members to understand—especially in families that have emphasized eating and rituals around when and how they prepare food. It is for this reason that many people dying in a hospital within the cure-based medical model have feeding tubes inserted for nourishment, even when they have specifically said they don't want them. In the hospital setting, dehydration is constantly treated with intravenous fluid lines in an attempt to keep the fluid balance in order. But people do not need to die in fluid balance. Unless you want these IVs, don't be pressured into accepting them.

Losing Bodily Functions

Later in the process of dying, you'll probably lose your ability to walk and care for yourself. You'll be using diapers and bedpans. Your friends and family must be prepared to deal with unpleasant sights and odors, especially if you're dying at home. You yourself may be repelled by what is happening with your body. It may help to remind yourself that you started this life in diapers, and there's a certain logic in your leaving it the same way. Have your caregivers pay close attention to keeping you clean, and accept what must be. Dying, like birthing, involves bodily fluids that are intense at first, but can be accepted as part of life.

A good example of this acceptance was provided by Mr. Van Normer, a patient who told me early in his hospitalization that he thought that being incontinent would be devastating. Surgery had shown that his cancer had spread too far to be curable. Within several months, he began losing control of both his bowels and his bladder. I explained to him that the hospital staff was very skilled at dealing with this situation and would keep him clean and comfortable. He sighed and shrugged. A short time later he said to me, "This incontinence is awfully embarrassing. But I guess it's just one more thing I have to accept." Because of the early discussions we'd had, he was prepared for what might happen and was able to deal with his feelings when the situation occurred.

When you're dying at home, all this can be difficult for your caregivers. Sometimes adult children have trouble with the idea that they're changing their parent's diapers; the old role is now dramatically reversed. You can help them recognize and laugh at the irony of the situation. If it remains difficult for them, they can enlist the help of health aides or others.

Breathing Problems

You may experience labored breathing, which can be scary both for you and for your caregivers. You can have awful sensations of suffocation. Fortunately, your doctor can prescribe morphine and other medications to relieve this sensation. If you're dying at home, your caregivers can be trained in the proper administration of these medications, including how to give injections. They will also have medical and nursing backup to help them manage this potentially difficult aspect of the dying process. Some of the people around you may have trouble watching injections being given and may need to leave the room. Don't be angry with them: everyone has a different threshold for such experiences.

Weight Loss or Swelling

You will also need to be prepared for the dramatic weight loss that usually accompanies dying. It can be frightening for your loved ones to see you looking emaciated; it can frighten you when you see yourself in the mirror. But remember, what your body looks like has never been the essence of who you are.

If you have advanced cancer, you may have severe swelling in your abdomen. Bowel and liver cancers, in particular, cause you to retain a large amount of fluid. Advancing tumors may disfigure your head, neck, or limbs. Again, you need to accept the circumstances as they occur.

If you believe in an eternal soul, focusing on that part of you can greatly help you face these bodily changes. One patient, an elderly woman with metastatic liver cancer, had a huge, swollen abdomen, swollen legs, and advanced jaundice. She told me that as her body was deteriorating she was able to project herself outside it and watch it as if she were a fly on the ceiling. She understood her self then as soul, since it was that self that left the body which, she believed, housed her soul. This conceptualization allowed her to relax and prepare for her actual dying.

Death

Last and greatest among the physical changes is death itself. In my experience, it is usually very peaceful. You'll probably slip slowly and gently into an unconscious state. In a relatively short time, you'll take in your last breath and then let it out. Most people die quietly, unconscious of anyone around them. Many make a final gesture, sometimes just a glance, toward the person who witnesses their final moments. Once it's clear that those final moments can be peaceful, you can move on to address other concerns with greater ease.

✦ STEP T ✦
Nurturing Your Body, Mind, and Spirit

It's important to relieve the tension, sadness, and heaviness of the dying process with humor, lightness of spirit, and pleasant diversions. What are your favorite hobbies? You have time now to indulge in them—depending, of course, on what they are. You won't get to do much mountain climbing at this point, but you can probably still manage a good game of chess or Trivial Pursuit. Do you love old Chaplin films or reruns of *Benson*? Make sure you've got a TV and VCR in your room, as well as your favorite tapes and TV listings. What do you enjoy reading—Agatha Christie mysteries, romance novels, Ray Bradbury? Indulge!

Don't underestimate the importance of music in your life at this time. Aside from the pleasure it brings, it can have a specific therapeutic effect. Many forms of music can serve this function. There are skilled music therapists and musicians who provide customized music for dying people in many communities across the United States. If there are no such musicians in your area, you can choose tapes that have a tranquilizing or spiritual effect on you. Do you love jazz? Rock? Opera? If you are up to it, make—or dictate—a list of your favorite songs and performers and ask friends or family members to bring you tapes of them. Such a task can be gratifying for someone who isn't able to play a major role in your care but still wants to help.

Help your friends and family create a comfortable, tranquil setting for you. Flowers, plants, and sunlight are cheering; so are photographs, pictures, and little statues—anything that makes your surroundings cozy and comfortable. One patient filled his room with his collection of model cars.

Physical comforts are especially significant at this time. Food is always important. Eat your favorites now, and if they don't cause uncomfortable symptoms, indulge all you want. One patient I worked with ate nothing but peanuts and beer in the last months of his life, and cheerily waved away the hospital staff who tried to make him eat more wholesome foods. Hospices, nursing homes, and even most hospitals nowadays are sensitive to the futility of strict diets when a patient is close to death, and if you're dying at home, you can call the shots. You may have to reassure overanxious caregivers that you're not hastening the end by eating what you want. Have the fun of gloating over them. *They* may have to watch their cholesterol, but *you* certainly don't! As I noted earlier, you may find yourself with less and less appetite, but when you do want food, have the food you enjoy.

Remember also that massage therapy can be very helpful as well. Ask for whatever care will make your body as comfortable as possible.

You also want to keep your mind calm. To help with this, you might want to review the discussion in Chapter 4 of how the mind creates disturbing repetitive thought patterns. Do all you can to prepare for a calm letting go, which requires a quiet mind. This is a time to let go of unrealistic expectations and to accept that whatever practical matters can be settled will be. Your main psychological goal now is to create a peaceful mind.

Of course, negative thoughts will enter your mind, just as they always have. Recognize them, work with them, and try, calmly and without self-reproach, to let them go. Professional counselors, clergy members, or friends can help you arrange your personal concerns at this time. I've found that simply reassuring my patients can be of enormous help to them in replacing negative thoughts with positive ones. "I assure you that everything will be fine," I'll say, or, "We will be with you, and you'll do wonderfully." These are things you can remind yourself too. It can also help to let your mind go to pleasant places—beaches, lakes, and other tranquil, sunny spots.

Family Fun

As you need comfort and support, so do your loved ones. They must find the care they need in their own lives from one another. But it can be hard for them to acknowledge their needs when yours are clearly more crucial. I'm often asked questions such as, How can I have fun while my father is dying? Yet, your family members *must* nurture their own physical, emotional, and spiritual lives in order to be helpful to you. Many people grow and make great changes in their lives as a result of their experiences with dying relatives or friends. Some alter their own views on living and dying as a result of seeing how loved ones have gone through the dying process.

One of the families I came to know in my work at the VA hospital was the family of Mr. MacGregor, consisting of four adult children, their spouses, and numerous grandchildren. Mr. MacGregor was a very reserved, elderly man, who held his emotions in until the last two weeks of his life. His family's attitude didn't help: everyone approached his imminent death with fear and denial. But over several weeks, thanks to the fine and persistent work of our staff psychologist, the family started to change. For instance, instead of continuing to shield the grandchildren from what was going on, the adults began bringing them to Mr. MacGregor's bedside.

The grandchildren's visits seemed to help him. Mr. MacGregor and I had talked a great deal about his fears, and those fears began to diminish. He used the affirmations I taught him, and because they helped him, he taught them to his family. Several days before his death, two of his children and several of his grandchildren talked to me about how his changed behavior had helped them. Since his dying was no longer a fearful process to him, they understood that they would not need to approach dying with the fears they had always assumed were inevitable.

I have also seen people realize their own spirituality as a result of experiencing a loved one's dying. Three days before slipping into a coma, one dying patient told his daughter that he was beginning to see a radiant light and hear beautiful sounds as he approached death. Though the daughter had not thought about her religion for many years, her father's experience convinced her that her own soul would live and that after her death she would visit lost relatives.

Remember, you and your loved ones can still have fun with each other. Watch a basketball game on TV together. Argue about the characters in your favorite soap opera. Perhaps more important, share old jokes—the old family stories that never grow stale because they're part of the history that binds you to one another.

At the same time, encourage your loved ones to go on with the rest of their lives, even as they're spending as much time as possible with you. Part of their work is to learn to live without you, as they soon must do. It is important that they continue getting fulfillment from their work and the usual pleasures of their lives. They need to see other friends and do the things they enjoy.

Unavoidable Anger

At times, you're going to feel angry—at fate, at God, at the people you love who are still healthy and will go on living after your death. This anger is normal, and you have to allow yourself to express it. Your friends and family need to understand that they shouldn't take it personally. In time, you'll move through the episodes of anger and back into your connections with them.

✦ STEP U ✦
Telling Your Story

One of the things you may want to do at this time is tell the story of your life, either by writing it down in a journal or by talking to others. Telling whatever parts of your story you choose to share helps put you in touch with your true feelings about your life. What did you do that you're proud of? What did you do that you regret? What was fun in your life? What was beautiful? What was sad? There are so many memories—your first kiss, your favorite childhood shirt, your first paycheck, the best vacation you had with your family. What was the best meal you ever ate, and where? What was the funniest joke you ever heard? The silliest thing you ever did? The biggest risk you ever took? Memories from the long-forgotten past can come up now, bringing with them pleasure, mellow sadness, a deep sense of connection with all the parts of the life you are leaving.

Telling your life's stories can also provide pleasure to those around you. It's amazing what even the closest friends and family members don't know about each other. By sharing memories of your life, you're giving those who love you more understanding of who you are and fuller memories of their own to cherish after your death.

It can also help to tell the story of the illness that is slowly taking you away from your present life. You probably feel cheated by life, and you have almost certainly been through a medical ordeal. Just being able to talk about that can help you find peace with your situation.

I learned from one of my mentors, Dr. N. Michael Murphy, about the importance of getting families to listen to a dying loved one tell the story of the illness during a family meeting (see Chapter 5, Step F). In my own work, I have expanded on Dr. Murphy's concept, and I encourage my patients to retell the story any time they wish. Simply talking to someone else about the specifics of the problem can help you feel less isolated.

Usually when I meet with someone facing an end-of-life situation, I try to get a brief life history. I ask patients where they grew up, what their families were like when they were kids, whether they were close to their parents, whether their childhoods were difficult, how many siblings they had, what their occupations were, what their marriages or other relationships were like, whether they had children, and so on. This serves a twofold purpose: the more information I have about a person's life, the better foundation I have for understanding that person's needs; equally, I find it helps the person to talk about it. For many patients, the shock of learning they have a serious illness turns out to be the most important moment of their lives. They often replay in great detail every conversation with doctors and relatives. Doing so provides great relief, helping them to both understand and accept what has happened to them, and to realize that some-one else understands and cares about the specifics of their disease and the battles they've waged against it. Now that the battle is over, it helps them to reexamine the story.

Once you have accepted that you are dying, your story—of your illness and of all the events of your life—takes on a different meaning. Telling it now helps you prepare for your dying and will help make that experience as peaceful and meaningful as it can be.

CHAPTER 10

Finding Peace

❧ STEP V ❧
Embracing Love as the Meaning of Life

*I*N ALL its many manifestations love can be the most important thing in your life right now. Take time to reflect on what love means to you, both in a personal sense and in a larger sense.

It can be very helpful to take time to think about the people you've loved in your life—friends, parents, children, lovers. If you're lucky, many of those you have loved are still around and can visit with you. It's important to be with these people, to express your love for each other. Too often people neglect to express love during the busy, preoccupied course of their lives.

I talked in Chapter 5 about the importance of dealing with unresolved issues. If you have been angry at a loved one, now is a good time to discuss the anger and to let go of it. People have doubtless let you down, as you have doubtless let them down, from time to time. Part of healing means facing this issue, talking it out, forgiving and being forgiven where that is needed.

It is also important to express your gratitude to your loved ones, especially your spouse, lover, children, close friends, and relatives. What have they done over the years that has helped you, pleased you, given you the strength to get through a rough time? Your expression of appreciation for them will be among the greatest gifts you will have ever given anyone. Express your love to people in whatever way you can, and receive theirs in return.

Not everyone you love will be present. Geography and time separate people. But all the love you have ever felt or received matters now. If you can't be in touch with some of the people you have loved, you can still recall the love and spend time thinking of it and feeling it. Your best friend in high school—whatever happened to him? Your closest sorority sisters—what silly, funny times you had together! These memories are precious, and though the time you spent with these people is long gone, the love isn't: it's somewhere inside you, and it's been a part of you all these years. Even the love you've had for pets is important: they are bonds with other creatures.

Sometimes you'll feel some regrets as you think about the people you've loved. There are often old hurts. Looking back, you may wish you'd spent more time with one person or been more attentive to another's needs. Don't be afraid of the regret, but don't exaggerate it. Ask yourself if you really did wrong or if you simply made choices based on the limitations of time and circumstance. Forgive yourself for the wrongs, and accept the limitations that were inevitable. You can't change past mistakes, but you can see if you learned anything from them. If not, you can accept their lessons now. Then try to let go of the regret: it no longer serves any purpose.

One poignant situation was that of Mr. Marx, a patient who was dying from advanced colon cancer. When I began working with him, I asked about his family. He told me that his only living relative was a brother he had quarreled with thirty years earlier. They had not spoken to each other since, and he had no idea where his brother now lived.

I suggested that we might do a computer search for his brother. Mr. Marx's eyes lit up. "It's been a long time," he said, "but I'd give anything to see Johnny and make it up with him before I die."

Unfortunately, my search kept coming up against roadblocks. By the time I was able to reach his brother, Mr. Marx had died. Yet the search itself helped him enormously. He had spent hours talking with me about the love he and his brother had felt for each other and the wonderful times they'd had together in their boyhood.

In thinking about the importance of love in your life, it is helpful to learn to appreciate the idea of unconditional love. Unconditional love exists without expectations or hopes that the person will return that love or do anything. Conditional love, in contrast, demands something in return for love: I love you because you can help me; I love you because I expect you to do something for me. Unconditional love is a pure experience that touches us by the beauty of its nature. This pure love is the physical expression of the bigger love we are all connected to.

A simple meditation can help you experience the power and beauty of pure love. Take a few moments each day to think of someone you can love unconditionally, without, at the moment at least, expecting or wanting anything from that person. Then you can experience an instant of peace. Begin by closing your eyes and concentrating on making your breathing slow and rhythmic. Picture a blank screen in the middle of your forehead. Then fill that screen with an image—a person, a pet, or even an experience that you can love unconditionally. Let the feeling that follows flow down your body from your head to your neck, your shoulders, arms, abdomen, and legs. Let the feeling fill you completely, and then expand to fill the entire room, the building, and then the world itself. Allow that feeling to completely fill your awareness and anything that flows from it as you grow to understand the power of unconditional love. This is one of the most marvelous meditations I know.

For people who believe in a larger reality, human love can be seen as the earthly expression of the love that governs the universe. Whether you think of it as God, a higher power, spirit, or in other terms, this love is often seen as the core of eternity. As Thornton Wilder wrote in *The Bridge of San Luis Rey,* "There is a land of the living and a land of the dead and the bridge is love, the only survival, the only meaning."

My own belief is that we come from love and return to love in order to learn its true essence. Love is the most powerful and important force in our existence. Connecting with this force can be an amazingly joyful experience. We can connect through love to an experience that goes beyond space and time. I've seen this connection transform dying itself from a process of fear to one of jubilation, becoming a vehicle for spiritual growth.

Many of the people I've worked with have found comfort in experiencing love for other people as a connection to a higher, loving force. One of my younger patients, Steve, had been married to his second wife for only eighteen months when he learned he was dying of pancreatic cancer. He had been abandoned by his parents when he was a child and had never believed himself worthy of love. Through his love for Susan, he began to love himself. In turn, this process helped him realize his love for his God. He told me that he felt connected to Susan, himself, and God through his deepest feelings, which he assumed came from his soul.

I saw a similar force in Mrs. Giovanni, an eighty-four-year-old woman I met when she was standing over the bed of her dying sixty-two-year-old son. As we got to know each other, she began telling me about her life. This was the second child she would see die. "I don't understand this," she said tearfully. "A mother isn't supposed to outlive her children. But I know the love I've shared with my children is the same love that exists in heaven and that the love is the connection between God, the angels, and all beings." With this faith, she did not fear her own death, knowing that she would be reunited with her children in heaven. "Put this in your book, will you, Doctor?" she asked me. "Maybe it will help some people."

Sometimes this love is experienced in a very mystical way. You may have heard of near-death experiences, when someone who is technically dead is revived and describes a journey toward a great light as well as feelings of joy and love emanating from an ocean of love and mercy. These experiences don't happen only to people who have technically died. Many of my dying patients have told me of such visions. They tell me of a peaceful, blissful state in which they fully experience what can only be called divine love. Experiencing this love puts these patients into a much more relaxed state. Some describe it as experiencing another world. Others call it entering into a new state of awareness.

One of my patients was a tough, streetwise man in his sixties, ironically nicknamed Little Johnny. He had advanced kidney disease and for many years had been coming to the hospital for dialysis. Eventually, as his health worsened, he decided to stop treatment. He realized that this meant he would probably die within two weeks, so he said good-bye to his close friends and his two cousins, the only family he had.

I was with Johnny when he began fading into a coma. He began to talk to me, very softly. "I'm going home," he said.

At first I thought he wanted to go back to his apartment, and I began to explain that this wasn't possible right now. But he continued to talk about going home, and I suddenly realized that it was I, not Johnny, who was confused. Staring into the distance, he told me that everything in his field of vision was beautiful, "colors of pure blue and love." He was looking at his place in the next world. His last words, before the coma overtook him, were "pure blue, pure love; I'm going home."

✶ STEP W ✶
Achieving Peace of Mind

Knowing that the plans you requested for peaceful dying are being respected, having your affairs taken care of, calmly saying good-bye to loved ones, and relaxing into the reality that all is in order and the way it has to be for now will greatly contribute to your peace of mind. All the steps in this book have been designed to help ensure this condition.

Peace of mind isn't some vague cliché: it's a relaxed, restful state in which grasping, regrets, and struggles are momentarily put to rest. It's a state you can work toward. I've seen a great difference in people who have chosen to get to this peacefulness, even when they've been able to remain in it for only a short time.

If you have been trying to reach this state but feel trapped by struggles and conflicts, it may be because you're still unresolved about something. Are there lingering feelings that you've wanted to talk about but felt you shouldn't? Maybe you need to figure out whom you can share such feelings with. You might have anger that, if expressed, could be hurtful to the person you feel the anger toward—someone you deeply love. Perhaps you need to express only *some* of your anger to that person and then to talk more fully to someone else about it—a counselor, clergy member, friend, or relative unconnected to the person involved. Find *someone* to talk with about whatever issue you have. Don't carry it around any longer.

You can use a variety of techniques to help you let go of your conflicts. To begin with, it helps to work at living in the present. This isn't as easy as it might sound. Most of us are usually fretting about the past and worrying about the future. Now it is time to release the notion that you can control everything. Fix what you can, and let go of the rest. The past is over: this is where you are now. Trust for a moment, if you wish, that everything happened as it was meant to: perhaps that will help you let go of the past.

You may need more techniques to help you achieve real peace of mind. It's important to be able to quiet your mind and create a reflective state. Looking and listening deep inside your-self, you can see and hear peace as a clear connection with the flow of life. To begin working on holding the experience of peace of mind, practice quieting your mind through a meditative or re-laxing technique (see Chapter 4, Step C). To work toward acquir-ing peace of mind, you need to create the right environment, as far away from noise and stimulation as possible.

A simple mind-quieting technique has helped many of the people I've worked with. Imagine that you are putting all the past problems that still bother you onto a raft docked on a river. Pile them all in—the specific issues and the vague ones. When all your concerns are in the raft, gently and lovingly push it away so that it floats down the river. Watch it drift away until you can't see it anymore. Then turn away from it.

You can do the same thing with concerns and fears for the fu-ture. Don't worry about deserting these concerns. If you really need to deal with them, when the time comes the raft will float back to you.

Creating this relaxed space for yourself will help you through the rest of your days, including the last one.

Dignity and Healing

Peace of mind, in some form, often comes to the person who is dying with dignity. Most people who are facing their dying begin, or continue, to ask questions about the meaning of their lives and the lessons learned throughout their journey. There is always time to look for what you can learn from your dying, rather than just waiting for death to occur.

People experience peace of mind in different ways. For some it's an occasional quiet, meditative movement, while for others it's a steady calmness that reflects the total acceptance of dying. How it occurs for you will be based on your own personality and life experiences. All the patients I've worked with, whatever their original anger, fear, or other emotional issues, have eventually managed to achieve some degree of peace of mind. Those who have spent their lives working toward a calm, balanced approach have tended to bring that approach to their dying. Those who have kicked and screamed throughout life have tended to continue doing so. Yet even they have been able to change at least a bit and move toward peace. The process of dying can be a great equalizer. It offers anyone who accepts it an opportunity to let go of the past and future and experience at least some degree of peace.

When you reach this peace of mind you are, in the deepest sense of the word, healing. Usually the word *healing* suggests getting better physically. That's not going to happen to you; you realize that by now. But deeper, more significant healing *can* happen at this time in your life. This is the kind of healing that begins when you allow life's hardships and joys to trigger a deeper examination of your life so that you can discover the individual lessons beneath the surface. You can experience healing when you accept, embrace, and learn those lessons, and realize that your life—the totality of your experience—has had a specific purpose.

Even if you die alone, or without the comfort of a special loved one, you can achieve healing and serenity. I have seen this happen many times. When you proceed through the process of dying, you have a great deal of time for reflection. Usually, toward the end, you will have many quiet days when you're unable to move from your bed and you're in a significant amount of physical and emotional discomfort. You have time to become aware of the meaning your life's experiences have had for you and of the wisdom you've gained from them. This in itself is a kind of healing.

As your life has been unique, so will your healing be. Though you may have learned great lessons from the healing you have seen others experience, ultimately your healing will be different because you are different. In the quiet of your mind and soul, reflect on the specifics that your life has taught you. Listen to your thoughts; be aware of the feelings that surface when you ask yourself these questions.

You don't need to have a happy life to find healing through dying. I have seen remarkable things happen in the dying days of people who lived alone, often on the fringes of society, angry and with no understanding from their lives of how to achieve peace. As time moves on, look, listen, and relax as best you can. Even a glimpse of peace of mind will open the possibilities of your creating more healing.

✦ STEP X ✦
Helping Plan Your Funeral or Memorial Service

I have found that many dying people take a lot of comfort from arranging the specifics of their funerals. Determining whether you want your body buried or cremated, whether you want a religious or nonreligious ceremony, and other aspects of the rituals that take place after your death involves your personal feelings and beliefs. Like the rest of your dying process, your funeral or memorial ceremony can reflect the choices you find most appealing. You can choose the text to be read at the ceremony and ask people to reflect on it. The conventional wisdom is that funerals are for the living, not for the dead; but many people want to know that the formal, public farewell to their life on earth will represent who they were. Even if family members and loved ones would like to see different events at the funeral and ceremony, they should honor your wishes.

The opportunity to help plan your funeral or memorial service is an advantage of your kind of dying over sudden death that many people think is preferable. A friend of mine remembers attending the funeral of her friend Carla, killed in a motorcycle accident, many years ago. Carla had been raised Catholic but had bitterly rejected the religion of her childhood. She was a lesbian, with no interest in marriage. The funeral Carla's parents arranged was traditionally Catholic—perfectly appropriate for someone who accepted that faith, but a far cry from anything Carla would have wanted. As my friend and Carla's ex-lover listened in horror, the priest announced that Carla was "now with her eternal bridegroom." The funeral had no relation to the person Carla had been; it related only to the person her parents wished she had been. Preparing your own funeral allows you to arrange for a service consistent with what you value.

Even if you're not going to have a formal funeral—for instance, if you want your body to be cremated or if you donate your body to a medical school—you can still be involved in preparing a memorial service or other farewell ritual. Often people who choose cremation want their ashes to remain in an urn in the home of a particular relative or friend. Others want their ashes scattered over a place that has been important in their lives.

I knew of a dying woman, a "party animal" all her life, who wanted to be cremated. Some of her happiest memories were of all-night parties. So she specified that her ashes be kept in an urn in the house of one of her sisters, who frequently had large, loud parties. Alive or dead, this woman wanted to be at those parties!

You may create an alternative, nontraditional service that best fits your character, or you may want to follow the pattern traditional to your religion or community.

My coauthor was close friends with another writer. When

Susan was dying of breast cancer, she asked Karen to write something to say at the funeral. Their friendship had been built around respect for each other's writing, and Susan wanted Karen's writing to be part of her service. For Karen, helpless to do anything to slow or cure Susan's disease, it was a comfort to know she could promise something that might help give peace to Susan's dying.

You might want to ask that the children in your life be included in the ceremonies. Allowing them to be a part of the funeral will help them become adults who have an honest and less fearful approach to dying. Also, as with adults, inclusion will help them express and deal with their grief at losing you. You and other adults can talk to the children now to see how comfortable they would be participating in or simply being present at your service.

By helping with your funeral preparations, you'll also be doing your loved ones a favor. Dealing with the details of a funeral can be difficult for people overwhelmed by grief. It is wise to contact a funeral director who will carry out prearranged requests for your funeral and your burial and thus reduce the need for family members to initiate arrangements at the time of your death. In addition, having someone who will arrange food and other necessities for the close family and friends after the service can ease the confusion immediately after your death.

❖ STEP Y ❖
Preparing Your Loved Ones for Their Bereavement

The people you love will suffer when they lose you. There's nothing wrong with this: grief, like death, is part of life. But there is much you can do now to help your loved ones prepare for the loss they will face.

To begin with, you can slowly, as best you can, let go of the people you love. As you begin to experience your own healing and peace of mind, you can convey this experience to your loved ones. You can let them know that you feel complete and peaceful and that dying at this time is all right. As you begin to do this, those around you may take their cue from you and begin their own process of letting go.

Letting go is also an acceptance of what must be—your dying. Many family members act as though their loved one will get better, even at the very end when it is clearly impossible. You can help them get rid of unrealistic expectations and the unhealthy belief that dying is a terrible thing.

If any of your loved ones are having difficulty admitting that you are dying, you can help them by firmly insisting that they acknowledge the truth, as you have. Further, you can help them prepare for the time after your death when they must both grieve and move on with their own lives. Talk to them about their feelings. Encourage them to continue talking with your palliative-care workers after your death if these people are still available. Explain to them that mourning tends to be greatest during the first nine to twelve months, and then it usually begins to subside. Mourning can take many forms. People may cry when thinking about the person they have lost. Sometimes the sadness takes the form of withdrawn silence. Some of your friends and loved ones may have moments of thinking they see you again when someone who looks like you walks by.

Signs of Depression

If your loved ones continue experiencing intense bereavement after the first year or so, they should seek professional counseling. One of the many support groups for bereaved people might be of help as well. And if they experience clinical depression, they need to seek professional help. Share this advice with them now.

Common signs of clinical depression include loss of appetite, a tendency to cry easily, lack of interest in things that used to be engaging, feelings of poor self-worth, agitation and panic, diminished libido, and a change in sleeping patterns. Anyone with such symptoms can get help from family doctors, clergy members, local mental health clinics, and hospitals.

Healthy Memories

You are not asking your loved ones to forget about you—not at all. You are reminding them that the greatest tribute to you is to allow their grief to transform itself into grateful memory, so that thinking of you creates less pain than happiness. The thought of you should bring memories of the time you have shared and the effect you have had on their lives. Such memories will always be tinged with sadness, and that's not a bad thing. But after a while, the sadness won't be the dominant emotion.

Just as you can learn much from your dying process, your loved ones can learn much by living through your dying and through their own bereavement. Those who witness your dying as positive and see you confront and diminish your fears of dying may be able to approach their own dying with greater balance and less fear. It is perhaps easier on those who believe that they will be reunited with you after their own deaths, but even loved ones without such sustaining faith can be enriched by the knowledge that you have lived well and died well and in the process made a difference in their lives.

❖ STEP Z ❖
Dying with Tranquillity

At this point, you have done a great deal of work to secure peaceful dying. Although it has doubtless been a difficult process, the rewards will be obvious. If you have used many of the preceding steps, you will be able to reflect now on the work you've done. You've expressed many feelings; you've learned many lessons. Now it is time to embrace tranquillity.

Even the most difficult physical and emotional end-of-life dying process can end well. The ways in which individuals achieve tranquillity differ greatly according to their personalities.

Mr. Weir came to the hospice unit where I worked with an advanced brain tumor. A very scared and bitter man, he was unwilling to talk to anyone. He would even throw medical staff out of his room. When asked how he was doing, Mr. Weir would growl, "Everything is fine!" and refuse to talk further. His family rarely visited him, and when they did, he treated them the same way he treated the staff. Yet even he softened in the end. Though he never really opened up to anyone, in his last three days Mr. Weir welcomed staff to sit with him at his bedside. The nonverbal communication between us showed me that he was dying with some tranquillity, but on his own terms. In some mysterious way, people have the opportunity to be guided toward tranquillity in their dying days.

Mr. Feathers provides a more clear-cut example of a person dying tranquilly. A delightful elderly man, Mr. Feathers was dying of metastatic lung cancer when I met him. Despite a constant supply of oxygen through his nose, he was severely short of breath—a situation that can cause a patient much panic and discomfort. Gasping for oxygen, the life source, is a particularly frightening and uncomfortable experience.

Mr. Feathers had fought long and hard to survive. Multiple surgeries, chemotherapy—he had used every available medical tool to fight for his life for many years. Shortly before I met him, he had accepted the inevitable and asked to be transferred to a hospice unit and given comfort care alone. When we first talked, he asked for my help. "I'm ready to move on. I'm not asking you to save my life," he said, "but when my breathing slows down like this, I'm so scared of suffocating."

The staff provided him with round-the-clock morphine, which eased his pain and somewhat lessened his respiratory difficulties. But during the last few days of his life nothing could fully relieve his breathing problems. Yet as he was fading into unconsciousness, he was able to smile at me. "Doc," he said, "I know we did the best we could with this dying thing." He closed his eyes, and remained unconscious, breathing shallowly but not with ease, until he died three days later. That smile, that ability to remove himself momentarily from his intense suffering, showed me what tranquillity could look like.

In my years as a doctor I've seen many people choose the time to move from their connection to this life into a state of tranquil acceptance. Those who have worked through the steps of communication, who have been ready to shift into a care mode of treatment, and who have struggled toward healing and peace of mind have been the ones best able to choose when to let go of this life by embracing tranquillity.

Above all, perhaps, an understanding of the centrality of love is the greatest aid to achieving tranquillity. When you can embrace the love you have experienced in your life, without clinging to it, you are most deeply in touch with the greater love that underlies all existence. One of the most tranquil and beautiful deaths I know of was not one I was involved with, but one described to me by my coauthor. Her brother Keith was diagnosed with lymphoma at the end of 1979. A strong young man in his early thirties, he fought the disease for nearly two years, but, slowly and painfully, the disease took over. In the months of his illness this shy, undemonstrative, insecure young man grew tremendously, understanding, through the love of his friends and family, how valuable a human being he had been. Through his illness, he and his loved ones got in touch with how deep their love for each other was. He grew spiritually as well, meeting with a lay brother from a nearby Catholic school.

On the last night of his life, Keith asked his exhausted wife to go home and get some rest; his brother Warren stayed with him in the hospital room. A psychic healer who had helped Keith throughout his illness was also in the room. Warren was in the bed, holding Keith in his arms, when suddenly Keith's breathing changed. He began to speak, his words like a litany of grace. "I love my wife, I love my daughter, I love everyone," he said, and repeated the words several times. Then he began again: "I love," and on that word, died. There was no fear, no pain, no terror—just an utter expression of love.

One of my own patients ended her life in a similar state of tranquillity. Mrs. Patterson was a fifty-five-year-old mother and grandmother who was my patient during several months of my medical internship. She had metastatic ovarian cancer, and I knew the chances of a cure were remote, but she and her family insisted on clinging to the hope that we could cure her. On her second admission to the hospital, several months after the first, Mrs. Patterson recognized me at once and told me how angry she was at the doctors who weren't curing her. I saw that she was in the very last phase of end-stage cancer. She and her family kept requesting consultations from different oncologists, desperately hoping to save her life. I tried talking to both Mrs. Patterson and her family about the likelihood that she was dying. No one would listen—there had to be a cure. I asked if she had worked on an advance directive, if she had talked with her family about unfinished issues. She persisted in refusing to address the reality of her imminent death. I was beginning to feel that I would never be able to reach her.

One morning as I was making rounds, Mrs. Patterson greeted me with a warm smile and asked me to sit down for a moment. "Dr. Tobin," she said, "I had the most incredible dream last night. I saw in my dream that everything was going to be all right when I leave this life. The figures I met in the dream showed me that I haven't been able to plan for my dying because I've been too afraid of it. And then when I woke up, I wasn't afraid anymore. Can you help me deal with my life in the best way possible?"

I was shocked at the transformation and delighted to work with Mrs. Patterson in her new resolve. Over the next month she worked with a local social worker skilled in end-of-life counseling. Though her family still resisted her dying, she pushed them into honoring her requests. All she wanted was to tell the people in her life how much she loved them and that she would miss them, but that her time in this life was ending. She no longer wanted any efforts made to prolong her life, only care that would contribute to her peaceful dying. She had her hospital room transformed into a beautiful space filled with flowers, quiet lighting, and music. Her oncologists made sure that she had adequate pain control, and her priest visited daily. She arranged her own funeral service and made certain she said good-bye to everybody who mattered in her life. Friends and relatives visited; even her cats were brought to her. A local musician came by frequently to sing with her. She made sure to thank everyone in the hospital, from the chief of staff to the cleaning woman.

Mrs. Patterson's transformation stunned the hospital staff, many of whom had known her for some time. They spoke of the lessons in living and dying that she was teaching them. I saw her shortly before she died. We spoke a while, and then I asked about the sudden, huge change after she'd had her dream.

She looked out the window into the bright sunlight. "In my

dream, I had the experience of being immortal—behind time and space and the mind that can understand this. From that moment I was no longer fearful." Mrs. Patterson died the next morning, surrounded by her family, her granddaughter holding her hand.

A tranquil death can happen to anyone. We need only to realize that the "great enemy" is in truth the ultimate friend.

The FairCare Health System and the Life Institute

As I've mentioned many times in this book, the current medical system in the United States is just beginning to examine ways to improve care of the dying. Doctors are primarily trained to focus on what they can cure and repair, so adjunct programs are needed to help bridge the gap between the public and those who provide end-of-life health care. I founded and developed the FairCare Health System—a set of model programs that can be copied—in order to provide the specific assistance people need with their dying. Clinical teams are already working within managed care organizations to provide integrated services in end-of-life care.

It is important to realize that the missions of the FairCare Health System and the Life Institute, as laid out in this appendix, are ideal models. They continue to develop in response to patient needs and demands. Indeed, end-of-life services will not become available to all patients until people start asking their doctors and health systems for such care. It will take time before all doctors and hospitals have end-of-life training and before education and counseling are available to all patients. Discussing these issues with your doctor or other medical professionals is one way to increase the likelihood that a program like FairCare will be available when you or a loved one really needs it.

- The FairCare Health System (FCHS) is a nonprofit, physician-based consultancy providing training for clinical teams in practical application of the twenty-six-step FairCare program to work with the public.

- FairCare Health System clinical teams are being placed into national medical care delivery systems via managed care organizations, health systems, and community organizations.
- Clinical teams comprise three practitioners—a doctor, a nurse, and a social worker—who provide education, counseling, advocacy, and coordination of services to people facing end-of-life situations.
- People facing end-of-life situations, and their families, will have the choice of utilizing the FCHS service, while maintaining all the medical options and practitioners.
- The FCHS clinical team will consult with treating physicians about pain management and advance directives.
- The FCHS delivers a comprehensive, mainstream medical end-of-life program by bridging the gaps between the person facing dying, the family and loved ones, the insurer, clergy members, and the health care practitioner.
- The Life Institute, a sister organization of the FairCare Health System, provides educational materials and programs to train health care workers in communicating with people facing end-of-life situations and with their families.
- The Life Institute provides a curriculum that enables health care workers to incorporate the material in this book.
- This curriculum is available to medical schools, residency programs, nursing schools, other health care workers, and clergy.
- The comprehensive curriculum is composed of didactic materials, clinical observation, and experiential workshops addressing individuals' fear of dying.

For more information about the FairCare program for peaceful dying, visit the website at www.faircare.org.

APPENDIX 2

Summary of FairCare Concepts

Step A: Recognizing Individuality of Disease, Individuality of Choice. Each person is an individual, who experiences disease uniquely. Once your treatment options have been clearly explained, it is your responsibility to decide on your own course of medical treatment and care. It is important not to relinquish your decision making to anyone else—neither doctor nor loved ones.

Step B: Confronting, Expressing, and Diminishing Fear of Dying. Fear of dying is deeply rooted in the difficulty of thinking, even briefly, about no longer existing in this life. Western culture encourages this fear by idolizing youth and hiding the reality of death and dying. Facing your fear can help you plan to secure a peaceful dying process and can enrich the living you will do until your death.

Step C: Slowing Down Time and the Mind. When you need to make crucial decisions, it's enormously helpful to slow down your mind, which tends to be filled with fast-paced, constantly changing thoughts and preoccupations. Taking ten or twenty minutes a day to quiet your mind will help you evaluate the choices available to you now. It will also help you focus on one decision at a time, rather than trying to deal all at once with the many issues that arise in an end-of-life situation.

Step D: Creating Positive Days. Each day should offer comfort and care to your body, mind, and spirit. To the extent that it is possible, you should do something that gives you pleasure and comfort. You need to think about what these things might be and ask others to help meet your needs.

Step E: Talking to Your Doctor—The Early Stages. Communicating your questions, fears, and desires to both your primary and your consulting doctors is crucial. The doctor in charge of your case will determine the specific nature of your medical treatments. You will want to get all the information available about your treatment options, their effects, and their side effects. Make sure that you have as many meetings with your doctor as necessary for you to understand thoroughly what is available to you.

Step F: Talking to Your Family. It's important to talk with your family members and loved ones about your illness and your concerns about how you will die. Discuss your treatment options and your decisions about specific treatments. Make certain that all your loved ones know what you want so that they will be advocates for you if you become unable to communicate. It is helpful to organize specific times for family meetings, if possible with a counselor who can help facilitate communication.

Step G: Coming to Terms with This Reality. The first thing you need to realize when you're given an end-of-life diagnosis is that you need time to adapt to it. You can easily be overwhelmed by events that may be in the future and that you may have no control over. Stick to what is real and true. Take one step at a time, and try to be as positive as you can be. Make a conscious choice to live each day as best you can.

Step H: Seeking Counseling and Support. You will need to seek out counseling from all your health care workers. Your primary-care physician, as well as other clinicians, may not be comfortable with giving you such counseling. You may have to search for the counseling resources in your community. It is worth the effort.

Step I: Selecting Advance Directives. Advance directives are written instructions placed in two main documents, the living will and the health care proxy. A living will documents your requests regarding future medical treatment. A health care proxy assigns someone to make your decisions if you become unable to do so yourself. Creating these documents early on in your illness can be helpful, but you will want to update them as your illness progresses. It's particularly important to discuss these documents with your primary physician; also, consider changing your standard living will to a crystal-clear do not resuscitate (DNR) will at the appropriate time.

Step J: Considering Other Practical Concerns. To prepare for your dying it's useful to arrange, in writing, all practical concerns related to your finances, personal affairs, where you will spend your last days, and any other important details that may need your attention. Doing this can help you to die with a settled mind.

Step K: Examining Spiritual Views on Living and Dying. Often someone facing the reality of imminent death begins asking questions about the meaning of life. The process of dying can be a great teacher, and exploring a spiritual understanding of life, however you define that, can help you find meaning in both your living and your dying.

Step L: Being Ready. When you reach the stage in an advanced illness when you are ready to die, you have accepted the fact that dying is a natural and inevitable part of living and you will probably no longer want to battle death aggressively. This is the time when you begin to let go of all your material and emotional preoccupations and to experience relaxation and closure.

Step M: Shifting to Care. You will now want to stop focusing on efforts to cure your disease and concentrate on dying in as much comfort as possible. The treatment plan must now shift from an acute, cure-based approach to a care-based one. The treatment philosophy is now palliative: that is, it should be geared toward making you comfortable and free of pain. You may choose to balance palliative with curative measures at any time.

Step N: Ensuring Family Support. Now that you have decided you want to focus on peaceful dying rather than on fighting your disease, you'll want to talk with your family and loved ones again. It's especially important that your health care proxy (see Step I) understand and agree to honor your request not to have your life prolonged by technical means. It will be helpful if everyone close to you accepts your wishes as well. Their acceptance will be better for your peace of mind and will make your proxy's job easier.

Step O: Talking to Your Doctor Again. Now that you have decided on palliative care alone, you must make this decision clear to your health care providers. You will most likely be the one to initiate the conversation with your doctor. You may want to change your living will at this time to include a DNR (do not resuscitate), if you have not done so already.

Step P: Dealing with the Suicide Question. It's quite common for people who have been given an end-of-life diagnosis to think about suicide, and dealing with the fear and despair that causes such thoughts can be a helpful part of coming to terms with dying. People often consider suicide because they fear dying in great pain or being abandoned. Knowing that pain can be stopped and that you won't be alone can help you consider choosing against suicide. FairCare, as a method of teaching how to secure peaceful dying, discourages suicide.

Step Q: Deciding Where to Die. It is probably best, if possible, to die at home—your own home or that of a loved one—so that you can be in familiar and comfortable surroundings without the regimens of a hospital setting. However, most people die in hospitals, and sometimes a hospital environment is the best or the only one available. There are many ways to make the hospital setting as comfortable for you as possible. If you live in a nursing home, you may choose to die there rather than in a hospital, and you should make your wishes known.

Step R: Getting Relief for Your Pain. Many medications are available that can completely relieve pain in virtually all situations. If you aren't getting sufficient pain relief, you can insist that your doctor contact a pain consultant and get the care that you need.

Step S: Dealing with Physical Changes. The process of dying brings dramatic physical changes. You and your loved ones should know what to expect. You will probably experience weight loss, lack of appetite, fatigue, and loss of bodily functions as your body slows down.

Step T: Nurturing Your Body, Mind, and Spirit. Physical, emotional, and spiritual nurturing are important elements in peaceful dying. As bodily changes occur, you must teach your mind to relax and let go. The process of dying takes place over weeks and months, and this time should be used to nurture your potential growth.

Step U: Telling Your Story. It is good at this time to talk to those around you about your life and about your illness. You may never have talked about much of your life before, and this is the time when doing so will be most helpful to you and most precious to those you leave behind.

Step V: Embracing Love as the Meaning of Life. Love as we experience it in our daily lives can be understood as an instance of an eternal, universal love to which we are all connected. Love is the most powerful force in the world. Approaching the process of dying positively and with an open mind may reveal to you that the greatest lesson anyone can learn from life is the nature of love. It is a great accomplishment to learn how to love yourself and to love others without expecting a conditional return. We come from love and return to love, in order to learn its true essence.

Step W: Achieving Peace of Mind. Peace of mind is a restful feeling in which struggle, grasping, and calculating are momentarily replaced by a sense that everything is in order. Knowing that your desire for peaceful dying is being respected, having your affairs taken care of, and saying good-bye to your loved ones can greatly contribute to your peace of mind. In this context, you are being healed, not in the sense of physical recovery, but in the personal growth and acceptance of all that your life has been.

Step X: Helping Plan Your Funeral or Memorial Service. You may want to arrange the specifics of your funeral or other ceremony with your family or loved ones. You can then make certain that the formalities of your death are what you want and reflect who you have been in this life.

Step Y: Preparing Your Loved Ones for Their Bereavement. Your loss will be a major event in the lives of those who love you. You can help them deal with this loss by talking with them about the bereavement they will face and helping them prepare for their grief.

Step Z: Dying with Tranquillity. As you prepare for your final days of conscious living, you can reflect on all the work you've done and the knowledge you've gained by securing your own dying process. A lot of struggle, sorrow, and joy are behind you, and it is time to settle into tranquillity. Even if your body is uncomfortable, you can find a way to relax into letting go of the will to stay in this life. You have done all you can to create a peaceful dying. You can now leave this life, filled with love and tranquillity.

Living Wills and Health Care Proxy Forms

The wording of living wills and health care proxies differs from state to state and may change over time. Rather than include forms for every state, this appendix shows samples from three states in different parts of the United States. These examples demonstrate the type of language these forms use and the issues they cover. Check with your doctor or health insurer about the proper documents for you. And remember, talking to your doctor, nursing home, and hospital about your wishes is extremely important.

The organization Choice in Dying maintains files of up-to-date documents for every state in the United States. You can access these documents on the organization's World Wide Web site, www.choices.org, or you can write to Choice in Dying, 1035 38th Street NW, Washington, DC 20007, (202) 338-9790

Aging with Dignity is an organization that provides the "Five Wishes" document, which includes living wills and health care proxy choices for thirty-three states. You can contact them through their Web site, www.agingwithdignity.org, or write Aging with Dignity, P.O. Box 1661, Tallahassee, FL 32302.

Connecticut Health Care Instructions

LIVING WILL

If the time comes when I am incapacitated to the point when I can no longer actively take part in decisions for my own life, and am unable to direct my physician as to my own medical care, I wish this statement to stand as a testament of my wishes.

I, _____
(name)

the author of this document, request that, if my condition is deemed terminal or if I am determined to be permanently unconscious, I be allowed to die and not be kept alive through life support systems. By terminal condition, I mean that I have an incurable or irreversible medical condition which, without the administration of life support systems, will, in the opinion of my attending physician, result in death within a relatively short time. By permanently unconscious I mean that I am in a permanent coma or persistent vegetative state which is an irreversible condition in which I am at no time aware of myself or the environment and show no behavioral response to the environment.

SPECIFIC INSTRUCTIONS

Listed below are my instructions regarding particular types of life support systems. This list is not all-inclusive. My general statement that I not be kept alive through life support systems provided to me is limited only where I have indicated that I desire a particular treatment to be provided.

	Provide	*Withhold*
Cardiopulmonary Resuscitation	_____	_____
Artificial Respiration (including a respirator)	_____	_____
Artificial means of providing nutrition and hydration	_____	_____
_____	_____	_____
_____	_____	_____

A sample living will currently utilized in the state of Connecticut.

INSTRUCTIONS

Florida Living Will

**PRINT THE
DATE**
**PRINT YOUR
NAME**

Declaration made this _____ day of _____, 19____.

I, _____, willfully and voluntarily make known my desire that my dying not be artificially prolonged under the circumstances set forth below, and I do hereby declare:

If at any time I have a terminal condition and if my attending or treating physician and another consulting physician have determined that there is no medical probability of my recovery from such condition, I direct that life-prolonging procedures be withheld or withdrawn when the application of such procedures would serve only to prolong artificially the process of dying, and that I be permitted to die naturally with only the administration of medication or the performance of any medical procedure deemed necessary to provide me with comfort care or to alleviate pain.

It is my intention that this declaration be honored by my family and physician as the final expression of my legal right to refuse medical or surgical treatment and to accept the consequences for such refusal.

In the event that I have been determined to be unable to provide express and informed consent regarding the withholding, withdrawal, or continuation of life-prolonging procedures, I wish to designate as my surrogate to carry out the provisions of this declaration:

**PRINT THE
NAME, HOME
ADDRESS AND
TELEPHONE
NUMBER OF
YOUR
SURROGATE**

Name: _____

Address: _____

_____ Zip Code: _____

Phone: _____

A sample living will currently utilized in the state of Florida.

State of New York
Department of Health

Nonhospital Order Not to Resuscitate
(DNR Order)

Person's Name _____

Date of Birth _____ / _____ / _____

Do not resuscitate the person named above.

Physician's Signature _____

Print Name _____

License Number _____

Date _____ / _____ / _____

It is the responsibility of the physician to determine, at least every 90 days, whether this order continues to be appropriate, and to indicate this by a note in the person's medical chart. The issuance of a new form is NOT required, and under the law this order should be considered valid unless it is known that it has been revoked. This order remains valid and must be followed, even if it has not been reviewed within the 90-day period.

A sample nonhospital do-not-resuscitate order currently utilized in the state of New York.

NAME: _____

M.R.#: _____

LOCATION: _____

DNR DOCUMENTATION SHEET #1
ADULT PATIENT WITH CAPACITY

Directions: This Documentation Sheet sets forth in consecutive order the steps that must be followed before writing a DNR ORDER for an ADULT patient with CAPACITY. Words that appear in the directions in all capital letters are defined in the DNR Policy. When completed, this sheet must be placed in the patient's medical record.

Step One

The ATTENDING PHYSICIAN must provide the patient with information regarding CPR and a DNR ORDER.

Attending Physician's Statement

I have provided to the patient information about his/her diagnosis and prognosis, the range of available resuscitation measures, the reasonably foreseeable risks and benefits of cardiopulmonary resuscitation for him/her, and the consequences of a DNR order.

_____

Signature of Attending Physician

_____

Date

Step Two

The patient must give oral or written consent to a DNR ORDER at or about the time the DNR ORDER is to be written. Oral consent must be given during hospitalization in the presence of two WITNESSES, one of whom must be on staff at the Hospital.

Witness's Statement

The patient has expressed orally in my presence the decision to consent to a DNR order, subject to the following conditions or limitations (if any): _____

_____

_____

Page one of a sample hospital do-not-resuscitate order currently utilized in the state of New York.

_____

Signature of Witness

_____

Print Name

_____

Title/Relationship to Patient

_____

Date

_____

Signature of Physician Witness

_____

Print Name

_____

Date

Instead of oral consent, the patient may choose to consent in writing to the DNR ORDER. Written consent must be signed by the patient and two WITNESSES. A copy of the written consent must be placed in the medical record.

Step Three

The ATTENDING PHYSICIAN must promptly do one of the following:
  a. issue the DNR ORDER, or issue the order at such time as any conditions specified in the patient's decision are met; or
  b. make his/her objections to the DNR ORDER and the reasons known to patient and either transfer the patient to another ATTENDING PHYSICIAN or refer the matter to the DISPUTE MEDIATION SYSTEM.

Indicate action taken: (check one)
_____ **DNR ORDER issued**
_____ **Patient transferred to another ATTENDING PHYSICIAN**
_____ **Referred to DISPUTE MEDIATION**

REMINDER: The DNR ORDER must be reviewed every three days, or sooner if there is an improvement in the patient's condition, and the review must be documented in the medical record.

Page two of a sample hospital do-not-resuscitate order currently utilized in the state of New York.

INSTRUCTIONS

Connecticut Appointment of Attorney-In-Fact
for Health Care Decisions

PRINT YOUR
NAME AND
ADDRESS

I, _____

(name)

_____

(address)

PRINT THE
NAME AND
PHONE NUMBER
OF YOUR
ATTORNEY IN
FACT

do hereby appoint_____,

(attorney-in-fact)

_____

(telephone number of attorney-in-fact)

to be my attorney-in-fact for health care decisions. If my attending physician determines that I am unable to understand and appreciate the nature and consequences of health care decisions and unable to reach and communicate an informed decision regarding treatment, _____

(attorney-in-fact)

is authorized to:

(1) Act in my name, place and stead in any way which I myself could do, if I were personally present, with respect to health care decisions as defined in the Connecticut Statutory Short Form Power of Attorney Act to the extent that I am permitted by law to act through an agent;

(2) Consent, refuse or withdraw consent to any medical treatment other than that designed solely for the purpose of maintaining physical comfort, withdrawal of life support systems, or withdrawal of nutrition or hydration.

PRINT THE
NAME AND
PHONE NUMBER
OF YOUR
ALTERNATIVE
ATTORNEY IN
FACT

If _____

(attorney-in-fact)

is unwilling or unable to serve as my attorney-in-fact for health care decisions, I appoint _____,

(alternative attorney-in-fact)

_____

(telephone number of alternate)

to be my alternative attorney-in-fact for health care decisions.

A sample health care proxy currently utilized in the state of Connecticut.

Florida Designation of Health Care Surrogate

PRINT YOUR NAME

Name: _____

          (Last)   *(First)*   *(Middle Initial)*

In the event that I have been determined to be incapacitated to provide informed consent for medical treatment and surgical and diagnostic procedures, I wish to designate as my surrogate for health care decisions:

PRINT THE NAME, HOME ADDRESS AND TELEPHONE NUMBER OF YOUR SURROGATE

Name: _____

Address: _____

_____ Zip Code: _____

Phone: _____

If my surrogate is unwilling or unable to perform his or her duties, I wish to designate as my alternate surrogate:

PRINT THE NAME, HOME ADDRESS AND TELEPHONE NUMBER OF YOUR ALTERNATE SURROGATE

Name: _____

Address: _____

_____ Zip Code: _____

Phone: _____

I fully understand that this designation will permit my designee to make health care decisions and to provide, withhold, or withdraw consent on my behalf; to apply for public benefits to defray the cost of health care; and to authorize my admission to or transfer from a health care facility.

ADD PERSONAL INSTRUCTIONS (IF ANY)

Additional instructions (optional):

A sample health care proxy currently utilized in the state of Florida.

Additional Resources and Reading

The best resources for an individual facing an end-of-life situation are almost always found within the local community. Ask your doctor, your hospital, and your health insurer about the services they can provide and refer you to. Check the local Yellow Pages and call the appropriate municipal and state government agencies. If you still have questions, the following national organizations may be able to answer them. Knowing how to contact these organizations is also useful if you wish to spend time advocating for or volunteering to help others who want to experience peaceful dying.

Academy of Hospice Nurses
32478 Dunford Road
Farmington Hills, MI 48334
(303) 432-5482

American Academy of Hospice and Palliative Medicine
P.O. Box 14288
Gainesville, FL 32604-2288
(352) 377-8900

American Association of Retired Persons
601 E Street NW
Washington, DC 20049
(202) 434-2277

American Association of Suicidology
4201 Connecticut Avenue NW, Suite 310
Washington, DC 20008
(202) 237-2280

American Hospice Foundation
1130 Connecticut Avenue NW, Suite 700
Washington, DC 20036-4101
(202) 223-0204

Children's Hospice International
901 North Washington Street
Alexandria, VA 22314
(800) 242-4453

Choice in Dying
1035 38th Street NW
Washington, DC 20007
(202) 338-9790

Deva House Children's Hospice
260 Summit Avenue
St. Paul MN 55102
(651) 602-0252

Hospice Association of America
519 C Street NE
Stanton Park
Washington, DC 20002-5809
(202) 546-4750

Hospice Education Institute
Five Essex Square
P.O. Box 713
Essex, CT 06426
(800) 331-1620

Hospice Nurses Association
5512 Northumberland Street
Pittsburgh, PA 15217
(412) 687-3231

Learning Center for Supportive Care
14 Orchard Lane
Lincoln, MA 01773
(781) 259-3110

National Association of People with AIDS
1413 K Street NW, Tenth Floor
Washington, DC 20005
(202) 898-0414

National Hospice Organization
1901 North Moore Street, Suite 901
Arlington, VA 22209
(703) 243-5900

National Prison Hospice Association
P.O. Box 941
Boulder, CO 80306
(303) 666-9638

Further Reading

Borysenko, Joan. *Minding the Body, Mending the Mind.* Bantam Books, 1987.
Bradshaw, John. *Homecoming.* Bantam Books, 1990.
Byock, M.D., Ira. *Dying Well: The Prospect for Growth at the End of Life.* Riverhead Books, 1997.
Carlson, Richard. *Healers on Healing.* Tarcher/Putnam, 1989.
Dossey, Larry. *Recovering the Soul.* Bantam Books, 1989.
Fisher, Louis. *The Essential Gandhi.* Vintage Books, 1962.

Frankl, Viktor. *Man's Search for Meaning.* Pocket Books, 1959.

Grollman, Earl. *Talking about Death.* Beacon Press, 1990.

Harper, Bernice Catherine. *Death: The Coping Mechanism of the Health Professional.* Southeastern University Press, 1977.

Jampolsky, Gerald G. *Love Is Letting Go of Fear.* Celestial Arts, 1979.

Kabat-Zinn, Jon. *Wherever You Go There You Are.* Hyperion, 1994.

Kübler-Ross, Elisabeth. *Death: The Final Stage of Growth.* Prentice-Hall, 1975.

Kübler-Ross, Elisabeth. *Death Is of Vital Importance.* Station Hill Press, 1995.

Kübler-Ross, Elisabeth. *To Live until We Say Good-bye.* Prentice-Hall, 1978.

Larson, Dale G. *The Helper's Journey.* Research Press, 1993.

Laskow, Leonard. *Healing with Love.* Harper San Francisco, 1992.

Levine, Stephen. *Who Dies?* Anchor Books, 1982.

Moody, Richard. *Life after Life.* Mockingbird Books, 1976.

Moore, Thomas. *Care of the Soul.* HarperPerennial, 1992.

Moreno, Jonathan. *Arguing Euthanasia.* Touchstone, 1995.

Moyers, Bill. *Healing and the Mind.* Doubleday, 1993.

Nuland, Sherwin B. *How We Die.* Knopf, 1993.

Peck, M. Scott. *People of the Lie.* Touchstone, 1983.

Peck, M. Scott. *The Road Less Travelled.* Simon and Schuster, 1978.

Reoch, Richard. *To Die Well: A Holistic Guide for the Dying and Their Caregivers.* HarperCollins, 1996.

Ring, Kenneth. *Heading toward Omega.* William Morrow, 1984.

Rinpoche, Sogyal. *The Tibetan Book of Living and Dying.* Harper San Francisco, 1993.

Rodgers, Carl. *On Becoming a Person.* Houghton Mifflin, 1961.

Sankar, Andrea. *Dying at Home: A Family Guide for Caregiving.* New York: Bantam Books, 1995.

Schachter-Shalomi, Zalman. *From Age-ing to Sage-ing.* Warner Books, 1995.

Stoddard, Sandol. *The Hospice Movement.* Vintage Books, 1992.

Taub, Edward A. *The Wellness Rx.* Prentice-Hall, 1994.

Webb, Marilyn. *The Good Death: The New American Search to Reshape the End of Life.* Bantam Books, 1997.

Acknowledgments

The writing and publication of this book are the culmination of many of my creative projects. I am extremely grateful to everyone who listened to and supported my creative vision throughout the various forms it has taken.

Jill Kneerim, my literary agent, artfully sold a book on peaceful dying when the marketplace told us it was crowded with books on the subject of dying. She combined the knowledge of a publishing executive with the skill of master martial artist in guiding the process to completion. I am extremely thankful to my editor, John Bell, who recognized the practical nature of this book, helped shape it and champion its message. I am grateful to everyone at Perseus Books who supported the FairCare vision and helped deliver it to the public. My coauthor, Karen Lindsey, graciously took on the project with integrity and personal charm. Her literary skills and ability to convey specific information in a friendly manner are obvious throughout the entire book.

I am indebted to Peggy Casey, an oncology nurse who immediately supported the FairCare concept and introduced me to her sister, Katie Tso. Katie, a talented publisher, editor, and writer, was kind enough to formally introduce this work to editor Thomas Grady. Mr. Grady, a leader in the world of publishing, recognized and embraced my original manuscript in very raw form, and for this I am deeply grateful. I will always credit Tom for getting me started as an author and being the godfather of this book.

Many thanks to Tom Monte for helping me write the proposal that sold this book and for writing many pivotal lines that summarized my concepts and were used in their entirety in the final manuscript. Special thanks to Tom for introducing me to Jill Kneerim and for helping me organize my thoughts in the fall of 1996 in Stockbridge, Massachusetts. Thanks to Sharon Silva and everyone at the Palmer and Dodge Agency. Thanks to Murray Caplan, Elliott Hoffman, George Stein, and Gil Karson for advising me on the legal issues involved in publishing. Cannon Rue Moore supported the vision in this work at an early stage.

Thanks to Joseph Fogel who assisted me by reviewing and editing my earliest manuscript with great skill and sensitivity. Pam Soccio did a superb job of typing and retyping the original manuscript, as did Ann Kotell later in the process.

Thanks to Len Belzer and Sandra Martin of the Paraview Agency for their support of my initial manuscript. Len's recognition of my early work was invaluable to the process of developing this book.

In developing the FairCare Health System, which enables health systems and managed-care organizations to provide the public with clinical teams trained in the FairCare concepts, I am indebted to Mr. John McDonald for all his endless work, selfless contributions, and evolving friendship. At the consulting firm of McDonald and Company I am indebted for all the work done on behalf of the FairCare Health System by Patrick Quirk, David Rossi, Alan Belvadere, and Linda Sharrad.

Within the V.A. Health System I am deeply grateful to Mr. Fred Malphurs, Dr. Joe Englehardt, Ms. Linda Weiss, Ms. Paula Hemmings, Ms. Bonnie Ryan, and Dr. Kenneth Kizer for all their support. Mr. Malphur's commitment to improving end-of-life care demonstrates, once again, how the V.A. Health System personnel respond to the needs of the human condition with courage and dignity. Dr. Bill Gorman recognized my work at its earliest stages and is personally responsible for the growth of the FairCare Health System. Ms. Karen Giles was helpful in developing the original plans for the FairCare Health System. I am indebted to Mr. Jim Conlon, a skilled and creative actuary at Milliman and Robertson, who supported my work from its inception and championed its entry in the managed-care area. Special thanks to Mr. Dan McCarthy at Milliman and Robertson, who supported the FairCare Health System at its very early stage. Mr. Bill Thompson graciously contributed time and energy to our initial business plans.

I am indebted to Dr. Dean Thompson and the Department of Medicine at the Stratton Veteran's Administration Medical Center, Albany, New York, for allowing me to be a part of their palliative-care team, and to Ms. Nancy Jane Batten, Dr. Peter Engel, Dr. Anna Rosen, Ms. Sandra Osborne, Dr. James Higgins, Mr. Mark Hahn, and the entire hospice/palliative-care team at the Albany VA, who helped me to visualize a new health system model for the dying.

Dr. Bill Popik, national medical director of Cigna Health Care, helped champion the FairCare Health System. Special thanks to Dr. Bob Kleinigger, Ms. Mary Ann McQuire, Dr. Manny Selva, Dr. Rachel Dennis-Smith, Dr. Victor Villagra, Ms. Joanne Puzzo, and everyone at Cigna Health Care who made the FairCare Health System possible.

Mr. Mike Christenson of the Allina Foundation recognized early my work and supported its development. Dr. Bob Greifinger, Dr. H.G. Bloom, Ms. Peggy Huddleston, Ms. Emily Squires, and Ms. Shirley Monzon supported my vision from an early stage.

Thanks to Dr. Michael Felder and Mr. Larry Trivieri, who reviewed the manuscript and offered sensitive evaluations of the major topics.

I am deeply grateful to Dr. Ira Byock for his guidance, support, and willingness to introduce me to the end-of-life community.

I cherish the support and love I received from my dear friend Mr. Robert Spall. Thanks for showing me the way.

I am indebted to Dr. N. Michael Murphy for his friendship, compassion, and willingness to teach me much of his common-sense medical wisdom in caring for the dying.

Dr. Howard Fogel, Ms. Karen Ranung, Mr. Ron Levine, Mr. Norman Toy, and Mr. Paul Yearwood have always been available and supportive friends.

I am grateful for the support and help of many other individuals. Dr. Bob McIntyre, Dr. Bernice Catherine Harper, Mr. David Becker, Ms. Mary Ann Boe, Dr. Carl Mindell, Dr. Larry Brown, Dr. John Wapner, Mr. Jeremy Sher, Dr. Greg Plonikoff, Mr. Michael Deluca, Dr. Gigi Hirsch, Mr. Peter Lucchese, Ms. Marilyn Feurgerson, Mr. Robert Huntley, Ms. Kathleen Quain, Mr. David Evans, Dr. Leonard Laskow, Mr. Leonard Marks, Dr. Maria Ramirez, Dr. Michele Strong, Dr. Daniel Callahan, Mr. Don Strong, Mr. Doug Schwartz, Mrs. Nancy Skuruik, Mr. David Schmuckler, Dr. Bill Kutscher, Mr. James Delgado, Dr. Hannah Hedrick, Dr. Joan Teno, Ms. Karen McKenzie, Dr. Michael Sedrish, Dr. James Plumb, Ms. Carolyn Cassin, Mr. Michael Vitez, Ms. Janice Schuster, Mr. David Purnell, Dr. Galen Miller, Ms. Sally Okun, Mr. Paul Brenner, Dr. Kate Christensen, Dr. Lawrence Flesh, Dr. Bob Babcock, Dr. Sheldon Solomon, Dr. Perry Fine, Mr. Tim Cousounis, Dr. Brownell Wheeler, Ms. Maggie Demars, Ms. Betse Cullen, Mr. James Towey, Ms. Genie Stranahan, Ms. Patty Baron, Mr. Stephen Kastner, Dr. Jack Stanley, Dr. Michael Gardner, Ms. Margie Ginsburg, Ms. Mary Strong, everyone at American Health Decisions, Ms. Sarah

Cronin, Mr. Ken Piazza, Ms. Shirley Chisom, Ms. Kathy France, Ms. Monica Verlardi, Ms. Sue Minardi, Mr. Joe Turton, Ms. Chris Glogowski, Ms. Mary Burbrick, Ms. Rita Ajmera, Ms. Laura Bareleski, Dr. Roberta Miller, Mr. Michael Finegan, Mr. Clyde Parkis, Ms. Darlene DeLancey, Dr. Jeffrey Fudin, Mr. Homer Thayer, Mr. Ronald Stockhoff. Ms. Janet Forlini, Dr. Bill Thomas and everyone at the Eden Alternative, Mr. Barry Smith, Ms. Barbara Ervin, Mr. Rick Lee, Mr. Marty Kuper, Ms. Connie Zuckerman, Ms. Carey Milne, Ms. Kathleen Meissner, Dr. Richard Holland, Lois Martin, Esquire, Mr. Christopher Lovelock, Mr. Warren Lindsey, Mr. John Sampson, Ms. Jacqueline Garrick, and the American Legion.

I am honored and humbled to stand in the long line of teachers whose work attempts to present values that can make daily living more meaningful. Many thinkers and writers have served as guiding lights to me: Elisabeth Kübler-Ross, Thomas Moore, Gerry Jampolsky, M. Scott Peck, and Kenneth Ring.

I have much fond love for my uncle, Professor Avram Holtz, who was the guiding light of my childhood. He showered me with love and showed me the joy of literature, poetry, and creative writing. Thanks to my dear mother, Helene, who always thought I should become a teacher rather than a doctor. Now, I am finally both.

I would like to thank my family and friends for all their kind support, tolerance, and love throughout my many creative projects that have culminated in the completion of this book. Families of those who try to blaze new trails are often asked to sacrifice more than their share. I am indebted to my wife and best friend, Robin, for her unlimited support in all my ventures, as well as all the extra work she willingly performed at home in my absence. My sons, Brian and Jeremy, supported my efforts and tried to understand why their father spent so many hours at his desk.

Much of what I have learned about living and dying comes from my firsthand clinical experience with thousands of people in varied settings. Caring for newborns, children, adults, and especially dying people of all ages has been a great privilege. Life, with its joy and suffering, mystery and technology, is lived and encapsulated in medical offices, hospital rooms, surgical suites, and treatment centers. I am grateful for, and respectful of, the relationships I have had with all my patients and their families over the last twenty years.

Index